Yohanna de Oliveira
Cássia Surama Oliveira da Silva
Hérika Wanessa Nóbrega Dantas de A.

Phytotherapy

Yohanna de Oliveira
Cássia Surama Oliveira da Silva
Hérika Wanessa Nóbrega Dantas de A.

Phytotherapy

Clinical and nutritional applicability

ScienciaScripts

Imprint

Cover image: www.ingimage.com

This book is a translation from the original published under ISBN 978-3-330-77233-5.

Publisher:
Sciencia Scripts
is a trademark of
Dodo Books Indian Ocean Ltd. and OmniScriptum S.R.L publishing group

120 High Road, East Finchley, London, N2 9ED, United Kingdom
Str. Armeneasca 28/1, office 1, Chisinau MD-2012, Republic of Moldova, Europe
Managing Directors: Ieva Konstantinova, Victoria Ursu
info@omniscriptum.com

Printed at: see last page
ISBN: 978-620-8-64140-5

SUMMARY

ABOUT THE ORGANIZERS

Yohanna de Oliveira

Master's student in the Postgraduate Program in Nutritional Sciences, with an emphasis on Clinical and Epidemiology Applied to Nutrition, at the Federal University of Paraiba (2016). Postgraduate in Clinical and Functional Nutrition from Faculdade Integrada de Patos (2017). Graduated in Nutrition from the Faculty of Medical Sciences of Paraiba (2015). She has experience in Clinical Nutrition, working mainly on the following topics: nutrigenomics, epigenetics, nutritional assessment, food consumption and obesity.

Càssia Surama Oliveira da Silva

Master's Degree in Nutritional Sciences, in the line of research in Clinical and Epidemiology Applied to Nutrition, from the Federal University of Paraiba (2014). Nurse in the Military Police Health Officers Cadre in the rank of 1st Lieutenant, working as Manager of the Urgency and Emergency Nursing Service at the General Edson Ramalho Military Police Hospital, Joâo Pessoa, Paraiba. Postgraduate in Workers' Health. Graduated in Nursing from Faculdade Santa Emilia de Rodat (1995).

Hérika Wanessa Nóbrega Dantas de Araùjo

Postgraduate in Clinical Nutrition - Metabolic and Nutritional Fundamentals, Gama Filho University (2010) and Postgraduate in Teaching and Management of Higher Education, Estàcio de Sá College (2017). Graduated in Nutrition from the Faculty of Medical Sciences of Paraiba (2007). She has professional experience in the areas of Clinical Nutrition and Nutrition and Aesthetics.

COLLABORATORS

Bianca de Sousa Fernandes

Bruno Rafael Virginio de Sousa

Géssica Gomes de Melo

Larissa de Fàtima Romao da Silva

Lusimere Almeida de Oliveira

Maria das Graças Silva

Ruanniere de Oliveira Silva

Stéfhani Eller de Freitas Pinheiro Florindo

Wlliane Silva Soares

DEDICATORY

We would like to dedicate this book to everyone who took part.

THANKS

Several people have contributed to the construction of this book, and we would like to express our thanks to them. First and foremost, we would like to emphasize our colleagues and collaborators who are authors, co-authors and responsible for the chapters, through their determination and determination, who have brilliantly fulfilled the task entrusted to them. Our special thanks go to the nutritionist Yohanna de Oliveira for her valuable collaboration in shaping the various chapters and for always being willing to help.

Finally, we would like to thank the publisher Novas Ediçôes Acadêmicas and its team for their partnership in this project and for the interest and attention shown to our work.

PRESENTATION

The book "Fitoterapia: Aplicabilidade Clinica e Nutricional" (Phytotherapy: Clinical and Nutritional Applicability) has an interdisciplinary content, contributing to the learning and understanding of various topics within the area under study.

This book is a collection of field studies, clinical cases and literature reviews derived from academic work on phytotherapy and nutrition, covering topics such as drug x nutrient interaction, the population's knowledge of the use of phytotherapics, the use of herbal teas for weight loss, the association of herbal medicines with nutritional therapy in wound healing, the importance of herbal medicine in pathologies such as diabetes mellitus and obesity, as well as presenting some of the most commonly used medicinal plants and classic concepts of herbal medicine.

The thematic axes addressed guarantee a broad discussion of results, thus encouraging, promoting and improving research that has sought to analyze the most diverse species of medicinal plants, their active principles and beneficial functions for the body.

The organizers aimed to divide each academic paper into specific chapters, so it consists of eleven (11) unpublished papers, i.e. those that have not been published or submitted to any conference or journal.

Finally, this book focuses on the applicability of phytotherapy and its importance in clinical and nutritional terms, with the aim of providing guidance to health professionals and expanding knowledge about the role of nutrients and the use of phytotherapics in the treatment of a wide variety of pathologies.

The organizers

CHAPTER 1

EVALUATION OF HEAT CONSUMPTION AND SOCIOECONOMIC AND ANTHROPOMETRIC PROFILES IN PRACTITIONERS AND NON-PRACTITIONERS OF PHYSICAL ACTIVITY IN TWO PARABANIAN MUNICIPALITIES

Hérika Wanessa Nóbrega Dantas de Araùjo[1] Yohanna de Oliveira[2]

Vanessa Fernandes Coutinho[3]

Daniel Granato[4]

1. Postgraduate in Clinical Nutrition - Metabolism, Practice and Nutritional Therapy - Gama Filho University;

2. Master's student in Nutritional Sciences, Federal University of Paraiba;

3. PhD in Food Sciences and Coordinator of the Postgraduate Course in Clinical Nutrition at Gama Filho University;

4. PhD in Food Sciences - University of São Paulo.

ABSTRACT: Tea consumption is an ancient practice of folk medicine, spread through family tradition and empirical knowledge as an aid to the treatment and cure of diseases. With this in mind, the aim of this study was to evaluate tea consumption and the socioeconomic and anthropometric profiles of people who practice and those who don't practice physical activity in two municipalities in Paraíba, Joâo Pessoa and Santa Luzia. A total of 300 individuals of both sexes, aged between 18 and 70 years or more, took part in this study, using an appropriate questionnaire to assess tea consumption and socio-demographic and anthropometric profiles. Descriptive and inferential bivariate statistics were used to analyze the data. A 95% confidence interval and 5% significance level ($p<0.05$) were adopted. The results showed statistically significant differences in some variables: What they turn to first when they feel ill (medicinal plants or traditional medicines), (age group ($p<0.001$), schooling ($p=0.02$) and income ($p=0.02$); simultaneous use of teas and medicines (Age group ($p=0.02$), schooling ($p=0.04$) and income ($p=0.02$); motivation for tea consumption (medical indication (Age group (0.03) and family tradition ($p=0.03$). In relation to the harmful effect of medicinal plants (age group ($p=0.03$) and income ($p=0.003$), the coefficients ranged from 0.12 to 0.28, suggesting a weak association between the variables. It was therefore concluded that there is a strong association between the prevalence among females and family tradition, as well as the population's lack of knowledge about the consequences of adverse reactions resulting from the concomitant use or substitution of medicinal plants and their derivatives (self-medication) with medicines.

Keywords: Folk medicine. Herbal medicines. Toxicity. Physical exercise.

1 INTRODUCTION

The use of medicinal plants as an alternative or additional treatment to pharmacological treatment has been growing and becoming more frequent every day (SILVA; HAHN, 2011), thus showing that it is still recognized as a popular medicine practice for the treatment and cure of diseases based on family tradition spread by successive generations in all cultures (BRASILEIRO et al., 2008; MARAVAI et al., 2011; FEIJÓ et al., 2012).

According to the World Health Organization (WHO), medicinal plants are "any plant that contains, in one or more organs, substances that can be used for therapeutic purposes or that are precursors of semi-synthetic drugs" (VEIGA Jr; PINTO, 2005).

Phytotherapics are medicines produced from these plants (FIRMO et al., 2011) and are defined according to the Ministry of Health's publication "Proposal for a National Policy on Medicinal Plants and Phytotherapeutic Medicines" as medicines whose therapeutically active components are exclusively plants or plant derivatives (extracts, juices, oils, waxes, etc.), and cannot include isolated active substances of any origin, nor associations of these with plant extracts. Phytopharmaceuticals are drugs (chemical compounds with therapeutic activities) extracted from plants or their derivatives (MINISTÉRIO DA SAÙDE, 2001).

Several factors have stimulated the increase in self-medication through the consumption of medicinal plants and their derivatives, contributing more and more to the growth of problems related to erroneous consumption: The emergence of new diseases that do not yet have adequate treatment, propagation of the concept of "natural", increases in the prices of conventional drugs (becoming less accessible the majority of the population, specifically rural dwellers); because they are low cost and easily accessible, (BRITO; DANTAS; DANTAS, 2009), difficulties related to access to public health services (ZARONI et al., 2004), the lack of supervision and regulation by the health authorities, the influence of the mass media, which markets products of plant origin and their derivatives with the expression "no contraindications" (FRANÇA et al., 2007), the use of medicinal plants, 2007), the use of medicinal plants associated with and/or replaced by synthetic medicines (MACEDO; OSHIIWA; GU ARIDO, 2007), a lack of knowledge about the toxicity of species (SILVA; DANTAS; CHAVES, 2010) and empirical knowledge acquired through cultural tradition and scientific knowledge conducted through clinical trials based on random data collection (ALEXANDRE; BAGATINI; SIMÔES, 2008).

However, contrary to popular belief based on the myth "if it's natural it doesn't hurt", they can cause reactions such as intoxication, nausea, mucous membrane irritation, edema (swelling) and even death, just like any other medication. However, it is believed that if certain precautions are taken, their use is favorable to human health, as long as the user has prior knowledge of their purpose, risks and benefits (BADKE et al., 2011; LOPES et al., 2010).

Considering the probable factors that have stimulated the growth of problems related to the erroneous consumption of medicinal plants and their derivatives, the toxic effects of the improper use of teas and their use in conjunction with medicines, and considering the differences in the socioeconomic and cultural level of the population and the purposes that drive such consumption, the aim of this study was to evaluate tea consumption and the socio-economic and anthropometric profiles of a sample of the population living in Joâo Pessoa - PB and Santa Luzia - PB, both practicing and not practicing physical activity.

2 MATERIAL AND METHODS

Type of study

The research is characterized as descriptive, exploratory, cross-sectional and quantitative.

Study population

The study sample consisted of 300 people, of whom 66 were men and 234 women. The sample was selected randomly. The study's inclusion criteria were: individuals living in the municipalities of Joao Pessoa - PB and Santa Luzia - PB, of both sexes included in the age groups imposed in the research (between 18 and 70 years or more), while the exclusion criteria were people living in other municipalities, children and adolescents of both sexes and under 18 years of age. Data was collected between November 2012 and July 2013.

Study site

The interviews differed in both cities in terms of where the data was collected. In Santa Luzia, they were carried out in Basic Health Units (UBS), home visits, in some stores and in a church in the city. In Joao Pessoa, data was collected in squares, churches, shops and gyms in different districts of the city.

Data collection instrument

The instruments used to collect the data were: G-Tech Glass 200 digital scale, duly calibrated and calibrated, installed away from the wall, with flat, firm and smooth surfaces, with a maximum capacity of 200 kg or mechanical anthropometric scale, with a capacity of 150 kg x 100 g division and a 28,5 x 37 cm, inelastic tape measure 150 cm long and accurate to 0.1 cm, for measuring hip and waist circumferences, Cescorf clinical adipometer (Plicometer), accurate to 0.1 mm and with a reading range of 80 mm, to measure skinfold thickness and an appropriate questionnaire containing 22 open and closed questions to assess tea consumption, socio-demographic data (gender, age group, marital status, schooling and income), as well as a form for recording anthropometric data such as weight (Kg), height (cm), waist circumference (WC), hip circumference (HC), waist-to-hip ratio (WHR) and triceps (TCA), biceps (BCA), supra-iliac (SIA) and subscapular (SSA) skinfolds.

Ethical considerations

With regard to ethical aspects, the assessments did not contain any information that would identify the individual or cause them embarrassment when answering. In addition, adults who agreed to take part voluntarily were included in the study, after obtaining verbal consent from the participants and signing the Informed Consent Form (ICF). In this way, the ethical principles of Resolution No. 196 of October 1996 of the National Health Council were respected throughout the process of carrying out this research.

Data analysis

The data was recorded in the form of a database in the statistical program SPSS (*Statistical Package for Social Sciences*) for *Windows*, version 20.0, and analyzed using descriptive and inferential bivariate statistics. For the descriptive procedures, absolute and relative data (frequencies and percentages), measures of central tendency (mean) and variability (standard deviation and minimum and maximum values) were presented. Statistical inference procedures were carried out using chi-square tests and Cramer's V coefficient, which identify associations between categorical variables. It should be noted that the qualitative nature of the variables submitted to inferential statistics was taken into account when choosing these tests. Finally, a 95% confidence interval and 5% significance level ($p<0.05$) were used to interpret the data.

3 RESULTS AND DISCUSSION

Assessment of the participants' socio-demographic profile

300 individuals from two cities in the state of Paraiba took part in the survey: Santa Luzia (63.0%) and Joao Pessoa (37.0%). The majority were female (78.0%), with only 22.0% male. As for age group, a considerable percentage of the participants in this study were between 21 and 30 years old and 31 and 40 years old, both with the same percentage of 21.0% and 20.0% in the 41 to 50 age group. The majority were married in both cities, both in Santa Luzia (45.5%) and Joao Pessoa (51.4%), according to the data shown in Table 1.

In terms of schooling, there were divergent percentages in the two cities: in Santa Luzia, the predominant level of schooling was incomplete secondary education (34.9%), while in Joao Pessoa there was a predominance of higher education (30.6%). From this perspective, the predominant income in Santa Luzia was between R$ 260.00 and R$ 780.00, while in Joao Pessoa it was above R$ 1821.00. The other percentages relating to schooling and income are also shown in Table 1.

In a study of the population of the municipality of Itaqui, carried out in pharmacies, a higher percentage of women (100%) were found to buy herbal medicines and medicinal plants. The authors justified the high percentage found for females by saying that, although women were the ones who bought the most herbal medicines and medicinal plants in pharmacies, this does not mean that men do not use them (ETHUR et al., 2011).

According to Ceolin et al. (2011), the predominance of women demonstrates the importance and responsibility of carrying out the propagation of knowledge and health care in the family between generations, using medicinal plants to do so.

Table 1. Socio-demographic profile of the study participants.

Variables	Subgroups	Saint Lucia		João Pessoa		General	
		f	%[a]	f	%[b]	f	%[c]
Sex	Male	39	20,6	27	24,3	66	22,0
	Female	150	79,4	84	75,7	234	78,0
Age range	18 to 20 years old	17	9,0	3	2,7	20	6,7
	21 to 30 years old	33	17,5	30	27,0	63	21,0
	31 to 40 years old	43	22,8	20	18,0	63	21,0
	41 to 50 years old	37	19,6	23	20,7	60	20,0
	51 to 60 years	28	14,8	19	17,1	47	15,7
	61 to 70 years old	19	10,1	14	12,6	33	11,0
	More than 70 years old	12	6,3	2	1,8	14	4,7
Marital status	Single	70	37,0	45	40,5	115	38,3
	Married	86	45,5	57	51,4	143	47,7
	Separate	18	9,5	6	5,4	24	8,0
	Viùvo	15	7,9	3	2,7	18	6,0
	No schooling	3	1,6	1	0,9	4	1,3
	Fund. Incomplete	32	16,9	14	12,6	46	15,3

	Fund. Complete	26	13,8	14	12,6	40	13,3
Education	High school incomplete	66	34,9	25	22,5	91	30,3
	Complete high school	18	9,5	16	14,4	34	11,3
	Incomplete university degree	18	9,5	7	6,3	25	8,3
	Complete university degree	26	13,8	34	30,6	60	20,0
	R$ 260,00 - 780,00	80	42,3	12	10,8	92	30,7
Income	R$ 781,00 - 1820,00	74	39,2	47	42,3	121	40,3
	More than R$ 1821,00	35	18,5	52	46,8	87	29,0

Legend: a Percentage calculated based on the number of participants from the city of Santa Luzia (n=189); b Percentage calculated based on the number of participants from the city of Joâo Pessoa (n=111); c Percentage calculated based on the total survey sample (n=300).

Assessment of the participants' anthropometric profile

As well as being analyzed in general, the data was analyzed according to the gender of the participants. BMI was found to be higher among male participants in the city of Santa Luzia; in Joâo Pessoa, it was the same. In all cases (males and females from Santa Luzia and Joâo Pessoa), the average BMI ranged from 25.4 to 26.9, which according to the WHO (1998a) nutritional status classification referred to in the Food and Nutrition Surveillance System booklet (MINISTÉRIO DA SAÙDE, 2004) is overweight.

WC measurements were within the normal range for men and women in both cities, although they were in the Iimitrophic ranges established by the criteria proposed by the Centers for Disease Control and Prevention (2002), in which a measurement of more than 102 cm for men and more than 88 cm for women is considered an independent risk factor for disease (MAHAN; ESCOTT-STUMP, 2010).

Interpreting the average WHR scores according to WHO (1998a) parameters, it was found that in the cities of Santa Luzia and Joao Pessoa, male and female participants in Joao Pessoa were outside the risk group for developing cardiovascular disease, a result contrary to that found for females in Santa Luzia.

The PCT, PCB, PCSE and PCSI measurements were found to be higher in females in both cities, as shown in Table 2.

Table 2. Anthropometric profile of the study participants.

Measures		Saint Lucia		Joao Pessoa		General	
		M±DP	Min-Max	M±DP	MinMax	M±DP	MinMax
BMI	M	26,9±4,8	19,5-41,5	25,5±3,8	14,2	26,3±4,4	14,2
	F	25,4±4,7	16,3-40,1	25,4±4,1	34,0	25,4±4,5	41,5
					16,0		16,0
					38,2		40,1
CC	M	96,4±14,1	70,0-131,0	90,5±11,4	62,0 107,0	94,0±13,3	62,0 131,0

	F	87,3±13,2	61,0-121,0	82,2±10,4	62,0 112,0	85,5±12,5	61,0 121,0
QC	M	102,3±9,9	84,0-127,0	98,6±6,2	83,0 115,0	100,8±8,7	83,0 127,0
	F	100,8±9,0	79,0-131,0	99,7±7,2	84,0 120,0	100,4±8,4	79,0 131,0
RCQ	M	0,93±0,07	0,79-1,11	0,91±0,08	0,741,07	0,93±0,07	0,741,11
	F	0,86±0,07	0,70±1,04	0,82±0,06	0,690,97	0,84±0,07	0,691,04
PCT	M	17,1±6,7	4,6-27,6	15,6±6,7	5,6-28,3	16,5±6,7	4,6-28,3
	F	19,9±6,9	3,6-43,6	20,6±6,4	4,6-35,6	20,1±6,8	3,6-43,6
PCB	M	10,1±4,8	3,6-24,6	11,8±5,9	3,6-26,3	10,8±5,3	3,6-26,3
F		13,8±6,7	3,6-39,6	16,1±6,9	2,6-34,3	14,7±6,8	2,6-39,6
PCSE	M	22,9±10,6	7,6-53,6	19,9±7,5	6,6-36,6	21,7±9,5	6,6-53,6
	F	23,2±9,4	6,6-46,6	21,5±7,1	2,6-40,6	22,6±8,6	2,6-46,6
PCSI	M	20,2±9,4	5,6-42,6	18,9±8,4	2,6-37,6	19,7±9,0	2,6-42,6
	F	22,7±8.9	6,6-50,6	22,2±7,5	7,6-41,6	22,5±8,4	6,6-50,6

Legend: a Percentage calculated based on the number of participants from the city of Santa Luzia (n=189); b Percentage calculated based on the number of participants from the city of Joao Pessoa (n=111); c Percentage calculated based on the total survey sample (n=300).

The formulas from the Durnin and Womersley (1974) protocol were used to calculate density (D). The Siri (1961) equation was used to calculate fat percentage (%F), while the Lohman (1992) protocol was used to interpret the %F results.

Initially, for density, an average of 1.04 was found for male participants and 1.02 for females. These values were found jointly for both cities, and separately in Santa Luzia and Joao Pessoa. Percentages of around 34% for females and 25% for males were observed in both cities, corresponding to an above-average percentage, which was therefore a high-risk fat percentage (obesity), according to the fat percentage table proposed by Lohman (1992). These data are described in Table 3.

Table 3. Assessment of fat density and fat percentage in residents of the cities of Santa Luzia and Joao Pessoa according to the gender of the participants.

Cities	Density		Fat %	
	Male	Female	Male	Female
	M±DP	M±DP	M±DP	M±DP
General (both)	1,04±0,01	1,02±0,01	25,06±5,78	34,31±5,34
Saint Lucia	1,04±0,01	1,02±0,01	25,44±5,72	34,15±5,61
Joao Pessoa	1,04±0,01	1,02±0,01	24,51±5,92	34,60±4,84

Evaluation of participants' consumption and knowledge of teas and medicinal plants

The subjects' use and knowledge of teas and medicinal plants was first assessed by asking them which teas they consumed. In Santa Luzia, the most prevalent responses regarding the types of tea consumed, in descending order of values, were: Boldo (85.7), erva cidreira (74.1%), camomila (60.3%), erva doce (56.6%), capim santo (51.9%), sabugueiro (49.7%), canela (38.6%), chá preto (31.2%), chá verde (24.9%), quebra pedra (18.5%), chá mate

(11.6%) and macela (11.6%). In Joao Pessoa, the teas most mentioned by the participants were: Boldo (74.8%), erva cidreira (65.8%), erva doce (55.0%), camomile (43.2%), capim santo (36.0%), châ verde (28.8%), cinnamon (24.3%), châ preto (16.2%), sabugueiro (10.8%) and châ mate (9.9%). Table 4 shows the teas mentioned by the participants.

Table 4. Presentation of the teas most mentioned by the participants.

Popular name	Scientific name	Saint Lucia		Joao Pessoa		General	
		f	% a	f	% b	f	% c
Avocado tree	*Persea spp*	10	5,3	3	2,7	13	4,3
Rosemary pepper	*Lippia sidoides*	17	9,0	6	5,4	23	7,7
Artichoke	*Cynara scolymus L.*	2	1,1	4	3,6	6	2,0
Bilberry	*Peumus boldus Molina*	162	85,7	83	74,8	245	81,7
Holy Grass	*Cymbopogon sympodialis*	98	51,9	40	36,0	138	46,0
Cinnamon	*Cinnamomum zeylanicum*	73	38,6	27	24,3	100	33,3
Chamomile	*Matricaria chamomile*	114	60,3	48	43,2	162	54,0
Carqueja	*Baccharis trimera*	3	1,6	4	3,6	7	2,3
Purple cashew	*Anacardium occidentale*	6	3,2	1	0,9	7	2,3
Green Tea	*Camellia sinensis*	47	24,9	32	28,8	79	26,3
Black tea	*Camellia sinensis L.*	59	31,2	18	16,2	77	25,7
Yerba Mate	*Ilex paraguariensis St. Hilaire*	22	11,6	11	9,9	33	11,0
Lemongrass	*Lippia alba*	140	74,1	73	65,8	213	71,0
Sweetgrass	*Pimpinella anisum L*	107	56,6	61	55,0	168	56,0
Espinheira Santa	*Maytenus ilicifolia*	12	6,3	5	4,5	17	5,7
Eucalyptus	*Eucalyptus globulus*	6	3,2	5	4,5	11	3,7
Ginger	*Zingiber officinale Roscoe*	10	5,3	5	4,5	15	5,0
Macela	*Achyrocline satureioides*	22	11,6	3	2,7	25	8,3
Stone breaker	*Phyllanthus niruri L.*	35	18,5	4	3,6	39	13,0
Quixabeira	*Bumelia sartorum Mart.*	4	2,1	1	0,9	5	1,7
Elderberry	*Sambucus australis*	94	49,7	12	10,8	106	35,3
	call						
Sene	*Cassia occidentalis*	18	9,5	2	1,8	20	6,7

Legend: a Percentage calculated based on the number of participants from the city of Santa Luzia (n=189); b Percentage calculated based on the number of participants from the city of Joao Pessoa (n=111); c Percentage calculated based on the total survey sample (n=300).

Analyzing the data in general (both cities), teas were also mentioned with a frequency of less than 5 participants. These were White tea (*Camellia sinensis* L.*)* (0.7%), red tea *(Camellia sinensis* L.*)* (1.3%), *hibiscus* (*Hibiscus sabdariffa Lineo*) (1.0%), melissa (*Melissa officinalis* L.) (0.7%), chayote (*Sechium edule*) (0.3%), pega pinto (*Boerhavia diffusa* L.) (0.3%), fedegoso (*Senna occidentalis* L.) (0.3%).) (0.3%), muçambê *(Cleome heptaphylla*) (0.7%), pepaconha (*Cephaelis ipepacuanha*) (0.3%), sete sangrias (*Cuphea carthagenensis*) (0.3%), orange peel (*Citrus sinensis*) (0.7%), roma (*Punica granatum*) (1.0%), guava leaf (*Psidium guajava*) (0.3%), chestnut leaf (*Terminalia catappa*) (0.3%), jalapa (*Convolvulus operculatus*) (0.3%), gogoia root (*Solanum capsicoides All*) (0.7%), skirt (*Kalanchoe *brasiliensis Cambess*) (0.3%), dill (*Anethum graveolens*) (0.7%), babatenon (*Pithecelobium avaremotemo Mart.*) (0.3%), mastruz (*Chenopodium ambrosioides L.*) (0.3%), banana leaf (*Musa sp.*) (0.3%), imburana (*Commiphora leptophloeos Mart.*) (0.3%), melindro (*Asparagus setaceus*) (0.3%), cana caiana (*Euphordia - Tiru -Calli*) (0.3%), colònia (*Alpinia zerumbet Pers.*) (0.7%), cana da india (*Canna indica*) (0.3%), cana do brejo (*Costus spicatus Sw.*) (0.7%), gypsy thorn (*Acanthospermum hispidum DC)* (0.3%), mulungu (*Erythrina mulungu*) (0.3%), mastic (*Schinus molle L.*) (0.7%), *basil* (*Ocimum basilicum*) (0.3%), *coriander* seed (*Coriandrum sativum*) (0.3%), *papaya* leaf (*Carica papaya*) (0.3%), laurel (*Laurus nobilis*) (0.3%) and olive (*Olea europaea*) (0.3%). Of the alternatives presented to the participants, only *horsetail* (*Equisetum arvense*) was not mentioned by any participant in either city.

Tea consumption was also investigated in terms of the weekly frequency of intake, the motivation for consumption and the professionals that patients went to for advice on the subject. With regard to weekly frequency, the majority of patients consumed between one and two times a week in both cities, 54.0% in Santa Luzia and 69.4% in Joao Pessoa, according to Table 5.

According to Gonçalves et al. (2011), in a survey carried out in the municipality of Volta Redonda - RJ, 270 participants stated that they used medicinal plants for a period of one week, indicating that the majority of users (77.8%) did not use the plants continuously.

Table 5. Evaluation of the frequency, motivation and professionals sought to clarify doubts about teas and medicinal plants.

Variables	Subgroups	Saint Lucia		Joao Pessoa		General	
		f	% [a]	f	% [b]	f	% [c]
Weekly frequency	Rarely	44	23,3	8	7,2	52	17,3
	1 to 2x a week	102	54,0	77	69,4	179	59,7
	3 to 4x a week	12	6,3	9	8,1	21	7,0
	5 to 6 times a week	5	2,6	7	6,3	12	4,0
	Daily	26	13,8	10	9,0	36	12,0
Reason to drink the cha	Healing diseases	115	60,8	51	45,9	166	55,3
	By habit or taste	59	31,2	52	46,8	111	37,0
	Medical indication	8	4,2	6	5,4	14	4,7
	Refer a friend	40	21,2	21	18,9	61	20,3
	Means of communication	7	3,7	7	6,3	14	4,7
	Aesthetics	7	3,7	17	15,3	24	8,0
	Family tradition	47	24,9	16	14,4	63	21,0
	Other reasons	12	6,3	1	0,9	13	4,3
Professionals who promoted guidance on the teas	Medical	29	15,3	16	14,4	45	15,0
	Pharmacist	4	2,1	10	9,0	14	4,7
	Nutritionist	13	6,9	22	19,8	35	11,7
	Nurse	11	5,8	5	4,5	16	5,3
	Others (friends and family)	143	75,7	69	62,2	212	70,7

Legend: a Percentage calculated based on the number of participants from the city of Santa Luzia (n=189); b Percentage calculated based on the number of participants from the city of Joao Pessoa (n=111); c Percentage calculated based on the total survey sample (n=300).

In this survey, the main reasons for consuming tea were to cure illnesses and for custom or taste in both cities, with each answer accounting for more than 30.0%. In the city of Santa Luzia, it is worth noting that another answer had a higher percentage than the one found in the city of Joao Pessoa. This was family tradition, cited by 24.9% of patients in the first city. With regard to the professionals sought for advice on teas, it was found that, in both cities, the source most cited by patients was friends and family, who were responsible for providing advice on teas and medicinal plants (Table 5).

Similar results regarding the motivation "to cure illnesses" were found by the following authors: Veiga Jr. (2008) observed that a considerable percentage of the population, over 90%, regularly used medicinal plants to cure their illnesses, 63.0% when there was some kind of discomfort or health problem; 12.6% preferred to use them for simpler cases such as colds and minor infections and only 1.4% of those interviewed in the survey used them as an alternative for terminal cases and Gonçalves et al. (2011) mentioned that 71% of the participants said they used or had used medicinal plants to treat some illness.

Also with regard to the consumption of teas by the participants, we sought to assess the justifications for using plants as medicines, the target population for such consumption and the place where the plants were purchased. At first, both in Santa Luzia and Joâo Pessoa, it was found that the participants turned to medicinal plants mainly because they felt their illnesses were relieved. As for the target audience of the teas, it was found that they were mainly adults, which was the same in both cities. However, in the city of Santa Luzia, another response stood out compared to the percentage found in the city of Joâo Pessoa: 35.4% of the participants in Santa Luzia reported that as well as adults and adolescents, children also consume teas (Table 6).

Table 6. Evaluation of the reasons for using medicinal plants, the people who use them and the place where the plants are bought.

Variables	**Subgroups**	**Saint Lucia**		**Joâo Pessoa**		**General**	
		f	% [a]	f	% [b]	f	% [c]
	Cheaper	8	4,2	5	4,5	13	4,3
Justification for	Likes	63	33,3	29	26,1	92	30,7
use of plants as		106	56,1	58	52,3	164	54,7
medicines	Disease relief Health benefits	53	28,0	34	30,6	87	29,0
	Teenagers	1	0,5	-	-	1	0,3

	Children and adolescents Children,-		- 35,4	1	0,9	1	0,3 28,7
People who use plants	adolescents and adults	67		19	17,1	86	
	Adults	105	55,6	86	77,5	191	63,7
	Children and adults	12	6,3	4	3,6	16	5,3
	Adults and teenagers	4	2,1	1	0,9	5	1,7
Location acquisition of plants	Backyard	46	24,3	29	26,1	75	25,0
	Neighbor's yard	28	14,8	21	18,9	49	16,3
	With relatives	18	9,5	17	15,3	35	11,7
	Mato	24	12,7	8	7,2	32	10,7
	Rooters	38	20,1	13	11,7	51	17,0
	Supermarket	128	67,7	73	65,8	201	67,0
	Specialty pharmacies	11	5,8	22	19,8	33	11,0

Legend: a Percentage calculated based on the number of participants from the city of Santa Luzia (n=189); b Percentage calculated based on the number of participants from the city of Joao Pessoa (n=111); c Percentage calculated based on the total survey sample (n=300).

It is common to observe tea consumption at all stages of life, the result of family tradition passed down through the generations for centuries. In view of the results found regarding the target audience, it is necessary to make some observations regarding the consumption of "teas" specifically by children, even though in this research it was not mentioned by the participants what age the children would be using the teas, and also the elderly adults.

In a study carried out with mothers of children under 4 months old in the municipality of Botucatu-SP, when asked about the most frequent reasons for giving water and tea to their children, 34.1% and 38.7% respectively answered that it was to quench the child's thirst and the second most frequent reason for drinking tea was the presence of colic in the infant (CARVALHÂES; PARADA; COSTA, 2007).

According to Table 6, in both Santa Luzia and Joao Pessoa, the most common places cited by the participants to buy tea and medicinal plants are supermarkets.

Zaroni et al. (2004), in a study to assess the microbiological quality of medicinal plants produced in the state of Paranà, found several pieces of evidence that are worth highlighting: The levels found of contamination by total aerobic microorganisms ranged from 2.0x102UFC/g to 1.7x107UFC/g, with 45.83% of the samples showing loads between 105 and 106UFC/g, the WHO (1998b) specification being a maximum of 5.0x107UFC/g for plant materials intended for use in the form of teas and infusions and a maximum of 5.0x105UFC/g for internal use. Mold and yeast contamination of the plant drugs analyzed ranged from 1.0x102 to 8.4x106UFC/g, with a higher frequency of samples with loads of 105UFC/g (36.11%), 95.83% presence of enterobacteria in almost all the samples, 22.22% of the samples analyzed counted the presence of enterobacteria, being related to the presence of Escherichia coli, a fecal coliform. Pseudomonas aeruginosa was found in seventeen samples (23.61%), a microorganism which, according to the authors, should be absent according to WHO specifications (1998b). Other Gram-negative bacilli found were: *E. agglomerans*, *E. cloacae, E. aerogenes*, *E. gergoviae*, *C. amalonaticus*, *K. rhino* and *A. hinshawii*. *Salmonella sp.* and *Staphylococcus aureus* were not found in the samples analyzed. Based on the authors' observations, these results show that the low microbiological quality of plant drugs found in the trade is not always due to negligence in marketing, and emphasize that the marked contamination may have originated in the production stages.

Pires and Araùjo (2011) mention the need for further chemical, pharmacological and toxicological studies before such products and herbs can be released for safe use. However, as these aspects are not always fully evaluated, specifically for native herbs in Brazil, it is necessary to take other criteria into account (traditional use and the coincidence of use of medicinal plants in different populations) so that they can be considered medicinal.

Participants were asked if they used any medication. It was found that most of the participants in Santa Luzia did not use medicines (54.5%), while in Joao Pessoa, the majority did use some medication (52.3%). They were then asked whether they prioritized medicinal plants or traditional medicines. In both cities, priority was given to traditional medicines. In a similarly high percentage of responses, 39.7% of respondents in Santa Luzia and 41.4% of participants in Joao Pessoa used plants and medicines together (Table 7).

According to Table 7, participants were asked about their doctor's reaction when they reported the use of herbal medicines. It was found in both Santa Luzia and Joao Pessoa that patients did not tell their doctors about their use.

Still on the subject of communication between doctors and patients, we asked the subjects what their main difficulty was in relation to the prescriptions made by doctors. The majority of patients in both cities cited reasons other than those given in the questionnaire, but did not mention which ones. Among the alternatives presented to the patients, it was found that in Santa Luzia the main difficulty was forgetting to follow the doctor's prescriptions (29.6%), while in Joao Pessoa it was the side effects of the medication (20.7%).

Table 7. Evaluation of the use of medicines, the priority choice when faced with a disease, the communication to the doctor about the use of phytotherapics, and the difficulties cited by the participants regarding the prescriptions of medicines prescribed by doctors.

Variables	Subgroups	Saint Lucia	Joao Pessoa	General

		f	% [a]	f	% [b]	f	% [c]
Use of medicine	Use (YES)	86	45,5	58	52,3	144	48,0
	No use (NAO)	103	54,5	53	47,7	156	52,0
Priority when sick	Medicinal plants	35	18,5	15	13,5	50	16,7
	Traditional medicines	79	41,8	50	45,0	129	43,0
	Both	75	39,7	46	41,4	121	40,3
Informing the doctor about herbal medicines	No information	137	72,5	68	61,3	205	68,3
	Approved	32	16,9	28	25,2	60	20,0
	Failed	5	2,6	3	2,7	8	2,7
	No opinion	15	7,9	12	10,8	27	9,0
Difficulties with doctors' prescriptions	Many medicines	14	7,4	8	7,2	22	7,3
	Forgetfulness	56	29,6	19	17,1	75	25,0
	Inconvenient hours	25	13,2	21	18,9	46	15,3
	Side effects	20	10,6	23	20,7	43	14,3
	Cost	14	7,4	9	8,1	23	7,7
	Other reasons	78	41,3	46	41,4	124	41,3

Legend: a Percentage calculated based on the number of participants from the city of Santa Luzia (n=189); b Percentage calculated based on the number of participants from the city of Joao Pessoa (n=111); c Percentage calculated based on the total survey sample (n=300).

Still on the subject of tea consumption, the participants' knowledge of the toxic effects of medicinal plants and phytotherapics was assessed, as well as the simultaneous use of teas and traditional medicines. In relation to the first question, in the city of Santa Luzia, the majority of patients believe that medicinal and phytotherapeutic plants are not harmful to health, as they are not natural (57.1%); however, in the city of Joao Pessoa, the majority of respondents believe that they can have harmful effects depending on the dose ingested (56.8%).

With regard to the simultaneous use of teas and traditional medicines, the majority of respondents reported not using them at the same time, a result found in both cities. As for the side effects of simultaneous use, the main responses in both cities were that they didn't usually use them simultaneously and that they never felt any bad symptoms or side effects. The third most cited answer by participants differed according to the city. In Santa Luzia, 24.9% of the respondents believed that the simultaneous use of teas and medicinal plants did not harm the patient; in Joao Pessoa, 16.2% of the participants said they did not know the side effects of the simultaneous use of teas and medicines, as shown in Table 8.

According to observations by Golçalves et al. (2011) about adverse reactions to the use of medicinal plants, they focus on the relationship between their occurrence and the popular thought that "if it's natural it can't hurt". A similar thought is mentioned by Defani et al. (2011), who state that even in natural products there is a risk of side effects which can lead to complications.

Medicinal plants and herbal medicines are characterized by being a complex mixture of chemical components that can act to benefit the body or act in a toxic way when administered simultaneously or as a substitute for allopathic medicines, and can interact with various drugs, causing changes in their plasma concentrations, reducing the activity of the drug and consequently losing its efficacy and/or safety, compromising health recovery and failure of therapy or progression of the disease (ALEXANDRE et al., 2008; VEIGA Jr; PINTO, 2005; VEIGA Jr, 2008).

Table 8. Evaluation of participants' perceptions of the harmful effects of herbal medicines, the simultaneous use of teas and medicines, and the effects of such use.

Variables	Subgroups	Saint Lucia		Joao Pessoa		General	
		f	% [a]	f	% [b]	f	% [c]
Medicinal plants and herbal medicines÷ Benefits	They're not bad for your health	108	57,1	48	43,2	156	52,0
	Yes, depending on the dose	81	42,9	63	56,8	144	48,0
Teas and remedies	YES, simultaneously	64	33,9	40	36,0	104	34,7
	NO simultaneous use	125	66,1	71	64,0	196	65,3
Side effects of simultaneous use	Yes, you have been informed	5	2,6	11	9,9	16	5,3
	More relief from illness	15	7,9	9	8,1	24	8,0
	No tea+ medicine	82	43,4	33	29,7	115	38,3
	No harm done	47	24,9	15	13,5	62	20,7
	No side effects	52	27,5	26	23,4	78	26,0
	You don't know how to answer	8	4,2	18	16,2	26	8,7
	Have you ever felt sick	1	0,5	-	-	1	0,3
	Depends on the tea and medicine	6	3,2	-	-	6	2,0
	Can cause effects	2	1,1	-	-	2	0,7
	Associate under guidance	-	-	1	0,9	1	0,3

Legend: a Percentage calculated based on the number of participants from the city of Santa Luzia (n=189); b Percentage calculated based on the number of participants from the city of Joao Pessoa (n=111); c Percentage calculated based on the total survey sample (n=300).

Physical activity assessment

This study also sought to assess the respondents' physical activity habits. In both cities, it was found that the majority of the subjects usually practiced physical activity, and the most practiced activity was walking, cited by 49.7% of the participants in Santa Luzia and 57.7% of those in Joao Pessoa (Table 9).

Table 9. Assessment of physical activity, specifying which activities and their frequency.

Variables	Subgroups	Saint Lucia		Joao Pessoa		General	
		f	% [a]	f	% [b]	f	% [c]
Activity physics	Not practical	74	39,2	23	20,7	97	32,3
	Physical activity	115	60,8	88	79,3	203	67,7
	Hiking	94	49,7	64	57,7	158	52,7
	Bodybuilding	23	12,2	22	19,8	45	15,0
	Aerobics	12	6,3	13	11,7	25	8,3
	Racing	2	1,1	1	0,9	3	1,0
	Pilates	3	1,6	-	-	3	1,0
Activities practiced		2	1,1	1	0,9	3	1,0
	Swimming Football	-	-	2	1,8	2	0,7
	Hydrogymnastics	-	-	3	2,7	3	1,0

	Skating	-	-	1	0,9	1	0,3
	Bicycle	-	-	2	1,8	2	0,7
	Kung fu	-	-	1	0,9	1	0,3
Frequency	No physical activity	70	37,0	22	19,8	92	30,7
Rarely		17	9,0	14	12,6	31	10,3
1 to 2x a week		16	8,5	15	13,5	31	10,3
3 to 4x a week		29	15,3	25	22,5	54	18,0
5 to 6 times a week		19	10,1	10	9,0	29	9,7
Daily		38	20,1	25	22,5	63	21,0

Legend: a Percentage calculated based on the number of participants from the city of Santa Luzia (n=189); b Percentage calculated based on the number of participants from the city of Joao Pessoa (n=111); c Percentage calculated based on the total survey sample (n=300).

With regard to the frequency of activity, the majority reported that they did it daily or 3 to 4 times a week in the two cities surveyed, as shown in Table 9.

Evaluation of tea consumption as a function of socio-demographic data

Prior to the inferential analyses, the socio-demographic variables were re-categorized in order to make it easier to compare the groups by delimiting them, increasing the sample size and distributing them proportionally. Thus, in the statistical inference procedures, the age group variable will be made up of the groups: (a) under 40 and (b) over 40. The schooling variable was recategorized into (a) up to elementary school, (b) secondary school and (c) higher education. The third socio-demographic variable, income, is now defined as: (a) from R$ 260.00 to R$ 780.00, (b) from R$ 781.00 to R$ 1820.00 and (c) above R$ 1821.00.

Initially, in order to assess the weekly frequency of tea consumption as a function of socio-demographic variables, the data was submitted to the Chi-Square test. The results showed that there were no statistically significant differences between the frequency of tea consumption and the participants' age, education and income.

However, statistically significant differences were found between the three socio-demographic variables for the questions of the use of any medication, what they turn to (medicinal plants or traditional medicines) as a priority when they feel ill and the simultaneous use of tea and medication. In these groups where the associations were statistically significant, they will be discussed in greater detail below. In relation to the malefic effect of medicinal plants, they only differed according to the age group and income of the respondents, and there were no differences in terms of their education level. The inferential values are shown in Table 10.

Table 10. Inferential evaluation of the weekly frequency of tea consumption, the use of medicines, what they resort to when they feel ill, the harmful effects of medicinal plants and the simultaneous use of teas and medicines according to the participants' age group, schooling and income.

Variables	Age range		Education		Monthly income	
	X^2	p	X^2	p	X^2	p
Weekly frequency of tea consumption	5,55	0,23	14,10	0,07	13,42	0,09
Do you take any medication	58,49*	<0,001*	10,43*	0,005*	6,80*	0,03*
Who do you go to when you're ill?	23,96	<0,001*	11,00*	0,02*	11,20*	0,02*
Harmful effects of medicinal plants	4,40*	0,03*	1,30	0,52	11,53*	0,003*
Simultaneous use of teas and medicines	5,19*	0,02*	6,23*	0,04*	7,07*	0,02*

Legend: * Statistically significant association.

Motivation for tea consumption was also assessed using inferential procedures. The results showed the following statistically significant associations: (a) consuming tea on medical advice differed according to age group; (b) consuming tea for aesthetic reasons differed according to the participants' schooling and income; and (c) consuming tea because of family tradition differed according to the participants' age group (Table 11).

Table 11. Inferential evaluation of motivation to consume teas and medicinal plants according to age, education and income.

Variables	Age range		Education		Monthly income	
	X^2	p	X^2	p	X^2	p
Healing diseases	1,80	0,17	0,78	0,67	1,64	0,43
You think it's nice	0,06	0,80	0,56	0,75	0,55	0,75
Medical indication	4,36*	0,03*	0,01	0,99	0,32	0,84
Referral from family	0,44	0,50	2,26	0,32	2,81	0,24
Means of communication	0,18	0,66	0,62	0,73	1,44	0,48
Aesthetics	0,97	0,32	8,66*	0,01*	10,92*	0,004*
Family tradition	4,71*	0,03*	0,005	0,99	0,15	0,92
Other reasons	0,03	0,85	0,31	0,85	1,03	0,59

Legend: * Statistically significant association.

With regard to the professional sought for advice on teas and medicinal plants, the following significant associations were identified: (a) the search for a medical professional differed according to the respondents' level of education and monthly income; (b) the search for a pharmacist differed according to income; and (c) the search for a nutritionist differed according to the participants' level of education and monthly income (Table 12). As for the other variables, no statistically significant associations were observed.

Table 12. Inferential evaluation of the professionals sought out for advice on teas and medicinal plants according to the age group, education level and income of the participants.

Variables	Age range χ^2	p	Education X^2	p	Monthly income X^2	p
Medical	0,88	0,34	7,08*	0,02*	6,31*	0,04*
Pharmacist	0,19	0,65	0,01	0,99	6,50*	0,03*
Nutritionist	2,10	0,14	8,42*	0,01*	7,69*	0,02*
Nurse	0,01	0,91	0,71	0,70	0,25	0,88
Friends/family	0,04	0,83	4,92	0,08	0,43	0,80

Legend: * Statistically significant association.

Evaluation of tea consumption according to age group

As shown above, some variables related to tea consumption were statistically significantly associated with the age group of the respondents. In this section, these relationships will be described in more detail, indicating which age group they were associated with.

These were (a) it was found that participants who consume teas by medical indication and by family tradition are over 40 years old; (b) participants who use medication are associated with being over 40 years old; (c) participants who primarily use teas and medication are under 40 years old; Similarly, it was found that those aged over 40 use either medicinal plants or traditional medicines separately; (d) it was found that those aged under 40 do not believe that medicinal plants can harm their health; and (e) that people aged under 40 use tea and traditional medicines at the same time. The percentages corresponding to these associations are shown in Table 13.

Table 13. Inferential evaluation of the motivation for tea consumption, use of medicines, what people turn to when they feel ill, harmful effects of medicinal plants and simultaneous use of teas and medicines according to the age group of the participants.

Variables	Subgroups	Under 40 f	%	Over 40 years old f	%
Consume tea on medical advice	Following medical advice	3	1,0	11*	3,7*
	No medical advice	143	47,7	143	47,7
	χ^2 (p); V		4,36 (0,03); V	=0,12	
He consumes tea as a family tradition	Yes, traditionally	23	7,7	40*	13,3*
	Not by tradition	123*	41,0*	114	38,0
	χ^2 (p); V		4,71 (0,03); V	=0,12	
Are you taking any medication?	Yes, he takes medication	37	12,3	107*	35,7*
	Does not take medication	109*	36,3*	47	15,7
	χ^2 (p); V		58,49 (<0,001);	V=0,44	
What you turn to when you feel ill	Tea and plants	15	5,0	35*	11,7*
	Medicines	52	17,3	77*	25,7*
	Both	79*	26,3*	42	14,0
	χ^2 (p); V		23,96 (<0,001);	V=0,28	
Harmful effects of teas	It's okay	85*	28,3*	71	23,7
	Depends on the dose	61	20,3	83*	27,7*
	χ^2 (p); V		4,40 (0,03); V	=0,12	
Simultaneous use	Make use of	60*	20,0*	44	14,7
	No use	86	28,7	110*	36,7*
	χ^2 (p); V		5,19 (0,02); V	=0,13	

Legend: * Statistically significant association.

Considering the statistically significant association between these variables and the age group of the participants, Cramer's V coefficient was calculated to estimate the strength of the association. For the variables "tea consumption", "professional used when ill", "harmful effects of teas" and "simultaneous use of teas and medicines", the coefficients ranged from 0.12 to 0.28, suggesting a weak association between the variables. However, for the variable "takes medication", a coefficient of 0.44 was observed, indicating a moderate association with age (Table 13).

Evaluation of tea consumption according to education level

Based on education level, the following conclusions were drawn: (a) people who consume tea for aesthetic reasons have higher education (complete or incomplete); (b) respondents who mentioned going to the doctor for advice have up to primary education; (c) those who go to the nutritionist have higher education; (d) participants who currently use some medication have up to primary education; (e) respondents who resort primarily to teas and medicinal plants have up to primary education; (f) people who make simultaneous use of teas and medicines have higher education; likewise, it was found that people who do not usually make simultaneous use have secondary education (Table 14).

Table 14. Inferential evaluation of motivation for tea consumption, professional sought for advice on tea, use of medication, what they turn to when they feel ill and simultaneous use of tea and medication according to participants' level of education.

Variables	Subgroups	Fundamental		Medium		Superior	
		f	%	f	%	f	%
Consuming tea for aesthetics	Yes, for aesthetics	4	1,3	7	2,3	13*	4,3*
	Not for aesthetics	86	28,7	118	39,3	72	24,0
	χ^2 (p); V			8,66 (0,01); V=0,17			
See your doctor for advice	Yes, look	21*	7,0*	15	5,0	9	3,0
	Not looking for a doctor	69	23,0	110	36,7	76	25,3
	χ^2 (p); V			7,08 (0,02); V=0,15			
See a nutritionist	Yes, look	6	2,0	12	4,0	17*	5,7*
	Don't look for a nutritionist.	84	28,0	113	37,7	68	22,7
	χ^2 (p); V			8,42 (0,01); V=0,16			
Are you taking any medication?	Yes, it does	56*	18,7*	52	17,3	36	12,0
	No use	34	11,3	73	24,3	49	16,3
	χ^2 (p); V			10,43 (0,005); V=0,18			
What you turn to when you feel ill	Tea and plants	23*	7,7*	19	6,3	8	2,7
	Medicines	40	13,3	53	17,7	36	12,0
	Both	27	9,0	53	17,7	41	13,7
	χ^2 (p); V			1,00 (0,02); V=0,13			
Simultaneous use	Make use of	31	10,3	35	11,7	38*	12,7*
	No use	59	19,7	90*	30,0*	47	15,7
	χ^2 (p); V			6,23 (0,04); V=0,14			

Legend: * Statistically significant association.

Cramer's V coefficient ranged from 0.13 to 0.18 for all these variables, suggesting a weak association between these variables and the participants' schooling.

Evaluation of tea consumption according to monthly family income

For the participants' monthly family income, the following associations were identified: (a) people who consume tea for aesthetics earn more than R$ 1821.00 per month; (b) those who earn more than R$ 1821.00 do not usually go to the doctor for advice on teas and medicinal plants, but instead go to the pharmacist; (c) those earning up to R$ 780.00 do not go to a nutritionist for advice on teas and medicinal plants; (d) respondents earning up to R$ 780.00 were associated with not using any medication at the moment, although they usually resort to medication as a priority when they feel ill; (e) participants earning up to R$ 780.00 believe that teas and medicinal plants are not harmful to health, while those earning more than R$ 1821.00 believe that teas and medicinal plants can have harmful effects depending on the dose in which they are ingested; and finally, (f) participants who use teas and medicinal plants simultaneously were associated with those earning more than R$ 1821.00 (Table 15).

Table 15. Inferential evaluation of the motivation to consume teas, the professional sought to advise on teas, the use of medicines, who you turn to when you feel ill, the harmful effects of medicinal plants and the simultaneous use of teas and medicines according to the participants' income.

Variables	Subgroups	Up to R$ 780,00		R$ 781,00 - R$ 1820,00		More than R$ 1821,00	
		f	%	f	%	f	%
Consuming tea for aesthetics	Yes, for aesthetics	4	1,3	6	2,0	14*	4,7*
	Not for aesthetics	88	29,3	115	38,3	73	24,3
	χ^2 (p); V			10,92 (0,004); V=0,19			
See your doctor for advice	Yes, look	17	5,7	22	7,3	6	2,0
	Not looking for a doctor	75	25,0	99	33,0	81*	27,0*
	χ^2 (p); V			6,31 (0,04); V=0,14			
Go to the pharmacist	Yes, look	4	1,3	2	0,7	8*	2,7*
	Not looking for a pharmacist.	88	29,3	119	39,7	79	26,3
	$\chi2$ (p); V			6,50 (0,03); V=0,14			
See a nutritionist	Yes, look	4	1,3	16	5,3	15	5,0
	Don't look for nutrition.	88*	29,3*	105	35,0	72	24,0
	χ^2 (p); V			7,69 (0,02); V=0,16			
Are you taking any medication?	Yes, it does	35	11,7	59	19,7	50	16,7
	No use	57*	19,0*	62	20,7	37	12,3
	χ^2 (p); V			6,80 (0,03); V=0,15			
What you turn to when you feel ill	Teas and plants	18	6,0	25	8,3	7	2,3
	Medicines	46*	15,3*	45	15,0	38	12,7
	Both	28	9,3	51	17,0	42	14,0

	χ^2 (p); V			11,20 (0,02); V=0,13			
Harmful effects of teas	It's okay	58*	19,3*	65	21,7	33	11,0
	Depends on the dose	34	11,3	56	18,7	54*	18,0*
	χ^2 (p); V			11,53 (0,003); V=0,19			
Simultaneous use	Make use of	29	9,7	35	11,7	40*	13,3*
	No use	63	21,0	86	28,7	47	15,7
	χ^2 (p); V			7,07 (0,02); V=0,15			

Cramer's V coefficient, like the results corresponding to the participants' schooling, ranged from 0.13 to 0.19, suggesting a weak association between the variables. The other coefficients are shown in Table 15.

4 CONCLUSIONS

The use of medicinal plants is a valuable resource as an aid in the process of health recovery, however, due to the influence of various factors, what should act in favor of a benefit, can lead to a worsening of health.

The results of this study show that there is a strong association between the consumption of medicinal plants and their derivatives (self-medication) and family tradition. However, the population was unaware of the adverse reactions caused by the concomitant use or substitution of medicinal plants and their derivatives (self-medication) with medicines.

Therefore, greater vigilance is needed in monitoring and regulating the use of medicinal plants and their derivatives in order to provide proven quality from cultivation to marketing.

The development of research in this area with an emphasis on adverse reactions and possible plant x plant and plant x drug interactions will help to enrich the knowledge of health professionals and students for better guidance for the population and in health care.

REFERENCES

ALEXANDRE, R. F.; BAGATINI, F.; SIMÔES, C. M. O. Interactions between drugs and herbal medicines based on ginkgo or ginseng. **Revista Brasileira de Farmacognosia**, v.18, n.1, p. 117-126, 2008.

BADKE, M. R. et al. Plantas medicinais: O conhecimento sustentado na pràtica do cotidiano populara. **Escola Anna Nery Revista de Enfermagem**, v.15, n.1, p. 132-139, 2011.

BRASILEIRO, B. G. et al. Medicinal plants used by the population assisted in the "Family Health Program", Governador Valadares, MG, Brazil. **Revista Brasileira de Ciências Farmacêuticas**, v.44, n.4, 2008.

BRITO, V. F. S.; DANTAS, I. C.; DANTAS, G. D. S. Medicinal plants used by the women's committee in the rural area of the municipality of Lagoa Seca - PB. **Revista de Biologia e Farmàcia**, v.3, n.1, p. 112-123, 2009.

CARVALHÂES, M. A. B. L.; PARADA, C. M. G. L.; COSTA, M. P. Factors associated with the situation of exclusive breastfeeding in children under 4 months, in Botucatu - SP. **Revista Latino-Americana de Enfermagem**, v.15, n.1, p. 62-69, 2007.

CENTERS FOR DISEASE CONTROL AND PREVENTION. **Basics about overweight and obesity**, 2002. Available at: <www.cdc.gov/nccdphp/dnpa/obesity/basics.htm>.

CEOLIN, T. et al. Medicinal plants: transmission of knowledge in the families of ecologically-based farmers in the south of RS. **Revista da Escola de Enfermagem da USP**, v.45, n.1, p. 47-54, 2011.

DEFANI, M. A. et al. Use of medicinal plants by diabetics in the Municipality of Goioerê - PR. **Revista Saùde e Pesquisa**, v.4, n.2, p. 223-231, 2011.

DURNIN, J. V. A.; WORSLEY, J. Body fat assessed from total body density and its estimation from skinfold thickness: measurements on 481 men and women aged from 16 to 72 years. **British Journal of Nutrition**. v. 32, p. 77, 1974.

ETHUR, L. Z. et al. Formal trade and profile of consumers of medicinal plants and herbal medicines in the municipality of Itaqui - RS. **Revista Brasileira de Plantas Medicinais**, v.13, n.2, p. 121-128, 2011.

FEIJÓ, A. M. et al. Medicinal plants used by elderly people diagnosed with diabetes mellitus to treat the symptoms of the disease. **Revista Brasileira de Plantas Medicinais**, v.14, n.1, p. 50-56, 2012.

FIRMO, W. C. A. et al. Historical context, popular use and scientific conception of medicinal plants. **Cadernos de Pesquisa**, v.18, p. 90-95, 2011.

FRANÇA, A. C. M. et al. Evaluation of Knowledge about Medicinal Plants among Students at Unileste, MG. **Revista Brasileira de Biociências**, v.5, n.1, p. 399-401, 2007.

GONÇALVES, N. M. T. et al. Popular tradition as a tool for implementing phytotherapy in the municipality of Volta Redonda - RJ. **Revista Brasileira de Farmàcia**, v.92, n.4, p. 346-351, 2011.

LOHMAN, T. G. **Advances in body composition assessment**. Champaign: Human Kinetics, 1992.

LOPES, G. A. D. et al. Medicinal plants: popular indications for use in the treatment of systemic arterial hypertension (SAH). **Revista Ciência em Extensâo**, v.6, n.2, p. 143-155, 2010.

MACEDO, A. F.; OSHIIWA, M.; GUARIDO, C. F. Occurrence of the use of medicinal plants by residents of a neighborhood in the municipality of Marilia-SP. **Revista de Ciências Farmacêuticas Bàsica e Aplicada**, v.28, n.1, p. 123-128, 2007.

MAHAN, L. K.; ESCOTT-STUMP, S. **Krause - Food, Nutrition and Diet Therapy**. 12ª ed. Rio de Janeiro: Elsevier, 2010.

MARAVAI, S. G. et al. Medicinal plants: perception, use and therapeutic indications of users of the family health strategy in the municipality of Criciùma-SC linked to PET-Medicinal Health. **Arquivos Catarinenses de Medicina**, v.40, n.4, 2011.

MINISTRY OF HEALTH. Secretariat of Health Policies - Department of Primary Care. **Proposal for a National Policy on Medicinal Plants and Herbal Medicines**, F ed., 2001.

MINISTRY OF HEALTH. Food and Nutrition Surveillance - SISVAN: **Basic guidelines for collecting, processing and analyzing data and information in health services**. Brasilia (DF), 2004.

PIRES, A. M.; ARAÙJO, P.S. Perception of risk and concepts about medicinal plants, herbal medicines and allopathic medicines among pregnant women. **Revista**

Baiana de Saùde Pùblica, v.35, n.2, p. 320-333, 2011.

SILVA, J. N.; DANTAS, I. C.; CHAVES, T. P. Plants used as abortifacients in the municipality of Bom Jesus-PE. **Revista de Biologia e Farmâcia**, v.4, n.1, p. 117128, 2010.

SILVA, B. Q.; HAHN, S. R. Use of medicinal plants by individuals with systemic arterial hypertension, diabetes mellitus or dyslipidemias. **Revista Brasileira de Farmâcia**, v.2, n.3, p. 36-40, 2011.

SIRI, W. E. Body composition from fluid spaces and density: analyses of methods. In BROZEK, J.; HENSCHEL, A. **Techniques for measuring body composition**. Washington: National Academy of Science, 1961.

SIRI, W. E. Body composition from fluids spaces and density: analyses of methods. In: Techniques for measuring body composition, Washington, DC: National Academy of Science and Natural Resource Council, 1961.

VEIGA Jr, V. F. Estudo do consumo de plantas medicinais na Regiao Centro-Norte do Estado do Rio de Janeiro: aceitação pelos profissionais de saúde e modo de uso pela populaçao. **Revista Brasileira de Farmacognosia**, v.18, n.2, p. 308-313, 2008.

VEIGA Jr., V. F.; PINTO, A. C. Medicinal Plants: Safe Cure? **Quimica Nova**, v.28, n.3, p. 519-528, 2005.

WHO World Health Organization. Obesity: Preventing and managing the global epidemic - **Report of a WHO consultation on obesity**. Geneva: WHO, 1998a.

WHO. World Health Organization. **Quality control methods for medicinal plant materials**. Geneva: WHO, 1998b.

ZARONI, M. et al. Microbiological quality of medicinal plants produced in the state of Paranà. **Revista Brasileira de Farmacognosia**, v.14, n.1, p. 29-39, 2004.

CHAPTER 2

SCARING ON VENOUS SORES USING *STRYPHNODENDRON ADSTRINGENS* AND FOODS THAT AID IN TREATMENT: A CASE STUDY

Géssica Gomes de Melo[1]

Ânderson Xavier Souza[1]

Yohanna de Oliveira[2]

Zianne Farias Barros Barbosa[3]

Maria das Graças Silva[4]

1. Nutrition undergraduates, Faculty of Medical Sciences of Paraiba (FCM/PB);

2. Master's student in Nutritional Sciences, Federal University of Paraiba;

3. Master in Food Science and Technology, Federal University of Paraiba;

4. Master's Degree in Natural and Synthetic Bioactive Products, Federal University of Paraiba.

ABSTRACT: Ulcers are chronic, progressive conditions which, if left untreated, can lead to serious complications, including necrosis, limb amputation and even death. They are located on the lower limbs, preferably in the internal malleolar region, and can be triggered by trauma, infection or venous insufficiency. Chronic cutaneous ulcerative processes are of great interest to health professionals who seek knowledge of the tissue repair process, The aim of this study was to evaluate the efficacy *of Stryphnodendron adstrigens* associated with diet therapy in the healing process of venous ulcers and specifically to characterize the patient with the ulcer in terms of nutritional status and the evolution of the wound during treatment, analyzing the healing time associated with diet therapy. This was a case study of a man with a chronic wound, of legal age, living in the municipality of Joâo Pessoa/PB, who was duly informed about the treatment. The ulcer sufferer was monitored for 331 days, between December 2015 and November 2016, and food consumption was assessed using the 24-hour food recall, anthropometric assessment and biochemical tests to record the patient's progress. The analysis was done by comparing and observing the patient's evolution. According to the results of the study, the existence of less invasive methods for tissue reconstruction in venous ulcers using *Stryphnodendron adstringens* and associated diet therapy was proven, which favored a reduction in physical and psychological suffering, as well as an improvement in the patient's clinical condition.

Keywords: Venous ulcer. Healing. Diet therapy. Barbatimao.

1 INTRODUCTION

Venous ulcers account for between 36.7% and 80.0% of all leg ulcers and their prevalence has been gradually increasing in line with the rise in life expectancy of the world's population and their most common etiological factor is venous insufficiency, triggered by venous hypertension (TORRES, 2016). It presents as an acute or chronic loss of skin continuity on an epidermal, dermal or mucosal surface, which may be accompanied by an inflammatory process. In the lower limbs, the three main types of ulcer are: arterial, neuropathic and venous, the latter with a prevalence of 80% of cases, its incidence has grown in line with the increase in life expectancy of the world population, and the prevalence has also been changing, being higher in people over 65 (ZUFFI, 2009).

Studies have been carried out on the impact of leg ulcers significantly affecting work productivity, generating disability pensions and normally restricting their activities of daily living and leisure. For many of these patients, venous disease means pain, loss of functional mobility and worsening quality of life (COSTA et al., 2012).

The most common cause of venous ulcers is venous insufficiency, and the conditions that predispose to this condition involve the process that will trigger venous hypertension, including deep vein thrombosis, multiple severities, edema, ascites, congenital anomalies, severe leg trauma, tumors, lifestyle, sedentary work, predisposition to standing or sitting for many hours without alternating with walking (DOUGHTY; WALDROP; RAMUNDO, 2000).

Wound healing is a complex event, involving the interaction of various cellular and biochemical components which occurs spontaneously, without external intervention, but which, when treated with artificial means, tends to occur more quickly and with better functional and aesthetic results. The possibility of speeding up healing and the complete reversal of skin damage, using chemical, medicinal or physical resources, has been the subject of investigation by numerous researchers (ZUFFI, 2009).

The use of plants for medicinal purposes, for the treatment, cure and prevention of diseases, is one of the oldest forms of medicinal practice in humanity. The concept established by the World Health Organization (WHO), considers that medicinal plants can be defined as any plant that has, in one or more organs, substances that can be used for therapeutic purposes or that are precursors of semi-synthetic drugs for use by the population of developing countries that depended on medicinal plants as the only form of access to basic health care (SOUZA et al., 2015).

According to Anvisa, medicinal plants can be considered as "any plant species, cultivated or not, used for therapeutic, phytotherapeutic purposes, or product obtained from a medicinal plant, or its derivatives, except isolated substances, for prophylactic, curative or palliative purposes", or as a traditional herbal product, which consists of "a product obtained exclusively from active plant raw materials, whose safety is based on traditional use and which is characterized by reproducibility and consistency of quality" (BRASIL, 2013).

According to Ferreira and Pinto (2010), indiscriminate use has often been influenced by the media's misinterpretation that it is a natural product, becoming a concern for health, since this can lead to cases of overdose, intoxication, interaction with other medicines/foods, as well as potential side and adverse effects.

According to Moura et al. (2016), in order to properly prescribe herbal medicines, it is necessary to master knowledge about medicinal plants such as: therapeutic effect, dosage, dosage, duration of treatment, form of presentation, adverse effects, interactions with medicines and food, as pharmacological and drug-nutrient interactions can lead to toxicity, ineffective treatment and nutritional deficiencies.

The human body needs energy and nutritional sources for the proper functioning of organs, cell repair, growth, development and regeneration of some damaged tissues, such as connective tissue and skin tissue (DINIZ, 2013).

According to Arcênio (2014), it is important to note that other non-nutritional risk factors should be assessed, such as age, chronic diseases, smoking, metabolic disorders, sepsis and medication (anti-inflammatory drugs), among others. In addition, it is common for nutritionists to come across patients with at least one of these factors, and the professional must be attentive to their nutritional status in order to prevent a worsening of the patient's condition.

Therefore, the general objective of this study was to evaluate the effectiveness of *Stryphnodendron adstrigens* (Barbatimao) associated with diet therapy in the healing process of venous ulcers and, as specific objectives, to characterize the patient with the ulcer in terms of nutritional status, and the evolution of the ulcer during treatment, analyzing the healing time associated with diet therapy.

2 MATERIAL AND METHODS

This is a case study with an evaluative approach, carried out through the follow-up of a patient living in the municipality of Joao Pessoa/PB, lasting 331 days, between the months of December 2015 and November 2016.

The sample consisted of one patient who underwent treatment using the tincture *of Stryphnodendron adstrigens* while cleaning the lesion with a solution of 0.9% saline solution diluted in the tincture in a ratio of 2:1. The damaged area was analyzed, considering its increase or decrease over the period under evaluation as a percentage.

Data was collected by taking photographs on a digital camera, before and during the treatment, in order to analyze the evolution of the wound. To analyze food consumption, a 24-hour food recall (REC24H) was carried out in order to characterize the patient's eating habits.

For the anthropometric assessment, a Plenna® digital scale with a capacity of 150kg and an accuracy of 100g was used. Height and knee height (KH) were obtained using an elastic tape with a capacity of 200cm and an accuracy of 0.1cm, according to the standards recommended by the World Health Organization (WHO, 2007).

The diagnosis of nutritional status was classified according to body mass index (BMI), calculated as the ratio between weight in kilograms (Kg) and height squared in meters (m), according to the WHO cut-off points (WHO, 2007) which establish underweight (BMI < 18.5 kg/m^2), eutrophy (BMI between 18.5 and 24.9 kg/m2), overweight (BMI between 25 and 29.9 kg/m2) and obesity (BMI > 30kg/m2).

The research project entitled "SICKNESS IN VENOUS SICKNESS USING *Stryphnodendron adstringens* AND FOODS THAT AID IN TREATMENT: A CASE STUDY" was submitted to and approved by the Ethics Committee of the Faculdade de Ciências Médicas da Paraiba (FCM/PB) under CAAE number 61515316.7.0000.5178.

Authorization was granted by signing the Informed Consent Form (ICF) for the use of images free of charge, preceded by a verbal explanation of the study's objectives and methods, in accordance with Resolution 466/2012 of the National Health Council, which deals with ethics in research with human beings.

3 RESULTS AND DISCUSSION

A 70-year-old male patient, recently diagnosed as pre-diabetic, denies smoking and drinking alcohol.

In the anamnesis, the patient reported that he had had the ulcer for four years, of venous origin, located on the left lower limb (LLL), and had previously been submitted to various topical treatments and analgesic medications, without obtaining any improvement in the lesion. According to the first nutritional assessment, the patient was diagnosed as being overweight, as shown in Table (1).

The ulcer had no flat edges or irregularities, the bed had no granulation tissue and there were sphacels, a large amount of serous-bloody exudate in the lower third of the MID, the malleolar region, edema, hyperemic adjacent skin and a complaint of intense pain.

Table 1. First anthropometric assessment carried out on 13/04/2016.

Anthropometric data	
Current weight (Kg)	74,5
Knee height (cm)	52
Height (m)	1,66
BMI (Kgm)	27,03
Theoretical Weight (Kg)	68
Nutritional status	Overweight

Initially, the patient was instructed to rest, elevating the lower limbs for 40 minutes in order to reduce the edema, and then a dressing was applied, following these steps: cleaning the wound with warm 0.9% saline solution with barbatim tincture, and this procedure was repeated until the end of the treatment.

As far as cleaning the lesion is concerned, this can be done with warm 0.9% saline solution to ensure effective cleaning and minimize the risk of additional trauma to the lesion (POLETTI, 2000).

According to Oliveira and Oliveira (2012), barbatim has an astringent function, a property that causes constriction of the tissues, reducing secretions, as well as precipitating protein substances that act to stop hemorrhages from small blood vessels or mucous secretions, so continuous and appropriate use allows the formation of a superficial crust on the affected areas.

Thus, the dressings were applied once a day for the first time, with a 24-hour interval between changes. After the 18th day, there was a reduction in exudate, no hyperemia and the presence of granulation tissue in the entire wound area (100%), as well as complete pain relief, allowing analgesic medication to be discontinued, which had previously been used daily.

After 60 days of treatment, the entire area of the lesion was still in the epithelialization phase and there was no exudate, edema or pain. After this period, there was no improvement in the patient's condition and it was necessary to investigate other factors. The REC24H test revealed a high intake of calories and refined foods, as shown in Table (2).

Table 2. 24-hour recall of venous ulcer patient before nutritional counseling.

Timetable/ Meals	Food	Homemade measure
08:00 Breakfast	Couscous	5 medium slices
	Whole milk	2 mugs full
12:30 Lunch		3 ladles full
		3 serving spoons full
		3 medium tablespoons
	Black beans White rice Cassava flour	2 medium thighs
	Stewed chicken Guarana soda	2 x 150ml glasses
15:00 Snack	Sweet Mary cookie	5 medium units 1 cup 200ml
	Soluble coffee	
18:00 Dinner	Hot dog Guarana soda	2 medium units 1 350ml can
22:00 Supper	Whole milk	2 x 250ml glasses

For a complete follow-up, it is extremely important to carry out a careful nutritional assessment, analyzing anthropometric parameters, including weight, height, BMI, biochemical and clinical tests, which should be carried out by a trained professional (SILVA; FIGUEIREDO; MEIRELES, 2007; AZEVEDO; ESCUDEIRO, 2009). Table (3) shows the results of the first biochemical test carried out on the patient.

Table 3. First biochemical test carried out on 13/04/2016.

Biochemical data	Result (mg/dl)	Reference values (mg/dl)
LDL cholesterol	124,0	Desirable: 130-159
HDL cholesterol	34,0	Low: <40
VLDL cholesterol	54,4	Up to 40 mg/dl
Total Cholesterol	212,0	Acceptable: 200-239
Triglycerides	272,0	High: >200
Glucose	119,0	Intolerant: 100-125

After gathering this initial data, it became necessary to carry out nutritional education, characterized by a strategy established by public policies on food and nutrition, which is considered an essential tool for promoting healthy eating habits in all age groups.

The nutritional guidance was based on recommendations for a higher intake of micronutrients, which act in intermediate metabolism and in the metabolism of certain organs. In general, they are converted in the body into more complex molecules that function as coenzymes, which cannot be synthesized and must be supplied through the diet. Inadequate intake of micronutrients can lead to a series of deficiencies or even hypervitaminosis (BRUG;

OENEMA; CAMPBELL, 2003).

A study of non-malnourished patients with pressure ulcers who were supplemented with arginine, vitamin A, vitamin C, vitamin E, copper, zinc, selenium and folic acid found that after 8 weeks the intensity and size of the wound decreased significantly (VAN ANHOLT et al., 2010).

It has also been advised to consume foods rich in vitamin C, which plays an important role in the synthesis of collagen, as well as in the formation of new blood vessels. Adequate levels of vitamin C help to strengthen healing, due to the antioxidant properties that help the immune system and increase iron absorption. Vitamin C deficiency impairs wound healing and has been associated with an increased risk of wound infection (FRAGA, 2015).

After 4 months of nutritional counseling, laboratory tests were carried out again in order to check for any changes in biochemical values, as well as a second assessment of nutritional status, as shown in Tables (4) and (5).

Table 4 - Second biochemical test carried out on 31/08/2016.

Biochemical data	Result (mg/dl)	Reference values (mg/dl)
LDL cholesterol	107,0	Desirable: 130-159
HDL cholesterol	37,0	Low: <40
VLDL cholesterol	28,6	Up to 40 mg/dl
Total Cholesterol	173,0	Acceptable: 200-239
Triglycerides	143,0	High: >200
Glucose	110,0	Intolerant: 100-125

Table 5 - Second anthropometric assessment carried out on 31/08/2016.

Anthropometric data	
Current weight (Kg)	70,0
Knee height (cm)	52
Height (m)	1,66
BMI (Kg/m^2)	25,4
Theoretical Weight (Kg)	68
Nutritional status	Overweight

Table 6. Third biochemical test carried out on 11/23/2016.

Biochemical data	Result (mg/dl)	Reference values (mg/dl)
LDL cholesterol	119,0	Desirable: 130-159
HDL cholesterol	39,0	Low: <40
VLDL cholesterol	26,2	Up to 40 mg/dl
Total Cholesterol	184,0	Acceptable: 200-239
Triglycerides	131,0	High: >200
Glucose	104,0	Intolerant: 100-125

Table 7. Third anthropometric assessment carried out on 11/23/2016.

Anthropometric data

Current weight (Kg)	Knee height (cm)	Stature (m)	BMI (Kg/m2)	Theoretical weight (Kg)	Nutritional status
68.7	52	1.66	24.93	68	Eutrophic

According to Armstrong et al. (2014), nutrition is an important factor in the repair of soft tissue injuries and wound healing, with certain nutrients proving to be more effective in the healing process. According to Silva, Figueiredo and Meireles (2007), the phases of the inflammatory process require specific nutrients which are fundamental in each phase of healing. In the initial inflammatory phase, vitamin K is used to synthesize prothrombin and coagulation factors VIII, IX and X, which are intended to reduce blood loss due to vessel damage and form a framework for fibroblasts to migrate to. The important nutrients at this stage are proteins, carbohydrates and indirectly, B vitamins, lipids, zinc, magnesium; collagen synthesis, in which amino acids, vitamin C and iron are used. In the remodeling phase, the process of maturation and stabilization of collagen synthesis and degradation takes place, giving the scar tensile strength. The most important nutrients in this phase are proteins, amino acids, carbohydrates, lipids, vitamins A, C and E, zinc and copper (SILVA; FIGUEIREDO; MEIRELES, 2007).

4 CONCLUSIONS

The application of the technique used in this study combined with diet therapy proved to be effective, providing a significant improvement in the patient's ulcer in all its characteristics, with a reduction in the size of the lesion, control of exudate, pain relief, reduction of edema and improvement in the patient's self-esteem, although this was not assessed using a specific instrument. Therefore, it should be noted that the appropriate choice of topical and diet therapy was of fundamental importance in facilitating and accelerating the healing process, minimizing discomfort due to the presence of the wound and certainly having a positive impact on the patient's quality of life.

REFERENCES

ARCÊNIO, C. M. **The importance of nutrition in the healing process.** 2014.

18f. Course Conclusion Paper (Graduation in Nursing)- State University of Paraiba, Campina Grande, 2014.

ARMSTRONG, D. G. et al. Effect of oral nutritional supplementation on wound healing in diabetic foot ulcers: a prospective randomized controlled Trial. **Diabetic**

Medicine, v. 31, n. 9, p. 1069-1077, 2014.

AZEVEDO, S. O.; ESCUDEIRO, C. L. Nutritional support in nursing: a literature review. **Revista de Enfermagem Atual**, v. 9, n. 50, p. 17-21, 2009.

BRAZIL. Ministry of Health. National Health Surveillance Agency.

Collegiate Board Resolution no. 13, of March 14, 2013. Provides for good manufacturing practices for traditional herbal products. Official Gazette of the Federative Republic of Brazil, Brasilia, DF, March 15, 2013.

BRUG, J.; OENEMA, A.; CAMPBELL, M. Past, present and future of computer- tailored nutrition education. **American Journal of Clinical Nutrition**, v. 77, n. 4, p. 1028-1034, 2003.

COSTA, L. M. et al. Clinical and sociodemographic profile of patients with chronic venous disease treated at health centers in Maceió (AL). **Jornal Vascular Brasileiro**, v. 11, n. 2, p. 108-113, 2012.

DINIZ, A. G. **Relevance of nutrition in the wound healing process**.

2013. 51f Federal University of Minas Gerais. School of Medicine. Collective Health Education Center, Lagoa Santa, 2013.

DOUGLAS, D. B.; WALDROP, J.; RAMUNDO, J. Lower-extremity ulcers of vascular etiology. In: Bryant, R.A. **Acutand Chronic Wounds: nursing management.** 2ª ed. St. Louis: Mosby, p. 265-300, 2000.

FERREIRA, V. F.; PINTO, A. C. Phytotherapy in today's world. **Quimica Nova**, v. 33, n. 9, p. 1829-1829, 2010.

FRAGA, M. S. D. C. B. **Influence of Nutrition on Surgical Healing**. 2015. 17f Course Conclusion Work (Degree in Nutritional Sciences) - Universidade Atlântica, Barcarena, 2015.

MOURA, A. S. C. et al. Knowledge about medicinal plants and herbal medicines: a study with nutrition students. **Revista Interdisciplinar**, v. 9, n. 3, p. 18-25, 2016.

OLIVEIRA, G. S. S.; OLIVEIRA, I. M. S. Barbatimao in the treatment of skin lesions. **Cadernos de Agroecologia**, v. 7, n. 1, p. 1-4, 2012.

POLETTI, N. A. A. **Nursing care for patients with chronic wounds: the search for**

evidence for practice. 2000. 237f Dissertation (Master's Degree in Fundamental Nursing) - Escola de Enfermagem/USP, Ribeirao Preto, 2000.

SILVA, R. C. L.; FIGUEIREDO, N. M. A.; MEIRELES, I. B. **Feridas: fundamentos e atualiz.ações em enfermagem.** 2ª ed. Sao Caetano do Sul-SP: Yendis Editora, 2007.

SOUZA, V. F. et al. A diagnosis of the study of medicinal plants in science teaching. **Cadernos de Agroecologia**, v. 10, n. 3, 2015.

TORRES, S. M. S. G. S. O. **Association of sociodemographic, clinical and care aspects in the quality of life of people with venous ulcers in primary care.** 2016. 115f Thesis (Doctorate in Health Sciences) - Health Sciences Center, Federal University of Rio Grande do Norte, Natal, 2016.

VAN ANHOLT, R. D. et al. Specific nutritional support accelerates pressure ulcer healing and reduces wound care intensity in non-malnourished patients. **Nutrition**, v. 26, n. 9, p. 867-872, 2010.

WHO. WORLD HEALTH ORGANIZATION. **Global age-friendly cities: A guide.** World Health Organization, 2007.

ZUFFI, F. B. **The care given to users with venous ulcers: perception of users registered with family health teams.** Master's dissertation, Ribeirao Preto School of Nursing, University of Sao Paulo, 2009.

CHAPTER 3

BENEFITS OF NUTRITIONAL THERAPY ASSOCIATED WITH THE USE OF BARBATIMAN (STRYPHNODENDRON ADSTRINGENS (MART.) COVILLE) IN THE CYCATRITION PROCESS OF WOUNDS: A REVIEW OF THE LITERATURE

Bianca de Sousa Fernandes[1]

Stéfhani Eller de Freitas Pinheiro Florindo[1]

Maria das Graças Silva[2]

1. Undergraduate student in Nutrition, Faculty of Medical Sciences of Paraiba (FCM/PB);

2. Master's Degree in Natural and Synthetic Bioactive Products, Federal University of Paraiba.

ABSTRACT: The aim of this study was to investigate the elements involved in the process of tissue damage, as well as to correlate the importance of applying nutritional support together with Barbatimâo (*Stryphnodendron adstringens* (Mart.) Coville) for the individual's tissue restoration. The purpose of the nutritional therapy is to protect against the spread of the pathology and the favorable development of the healing process aided by the administration of Barbatimâo. Among the factors that favor the injury process, malnutrition and vitamin and mineral deficiencies stand out. Studies have found the effectiveness of carbohydrates, proteins, lipids, vitamin C (ascorbic acid), zinc, arginine and vitamin A as fundamental in tissue restoration, however, there are few studies related to the use of tocopherol (vitamin E), vitamin D, B vitamins and glutamine, thus suggesting that more studies should be carried out emphasizing these nutrients in the wound healing process. It was therefore concluded that the use of the active principles of Barbatimâo (*Stryphnodendron adstringens* (Mart.) Coville) are effective for effective healing, demonstrating that the role of nutrients and Barbatimâo in the healing process is to slow down the progression time of healing, provide energy for the process and act to maintain the appropriate state of hydration to improve the results of healing.

Keywords: Wounds. Nutrients. Healing. Nutrition. Barbatimâo.

1 INTRODUCTION

The wound healing process consists of dynamic repair and cell regeneration, involving biochemical and physiological phenomena, in which the injured tissue is re-covered and replaced by new tissue. This process is divided into five stages, which consist of: the coagulation stage, inflammation, proliferation, wound contraction and remodeling, it is worth noting that these stages will coincide and occur simultaneously (ORGILL; DEMLING, 1988).

In order to strengthen and speed up the patient's recovery, it is necessary to clarify the care and importance of maintaining nutritional and emotional balance, periodic dressings and hygiene care, thus enabling successful tissue healing (DEALEY, 2008).

In addition to the points mentioned above, the use of herbal substances combined with an appropriate diet can not only be an adjunct to treatment, but can also be the main treatment, speeding up the healing process and even preventing future injuries. Although herbal practices are considered by many to be non-scientific, but rather popular, techniques, in recent years studies have shown that their use and *effectiveness* in tissue regeneration processes has expanded (MARTINS et al., 2003).

Barbatimao (*Stryphnodendron adstringens* (Mart.) Coville) has been widely used to treat wounds due to its composition of tannins, the active ingredient that gives it an astringent action, as well as anti-inflammatory, analgesic and gastric mucosa-protecting properties (MARTINS et al., 2003; BEZERRA et al., 2002).

In this sense, it is essential to assess and monitor the nutritional status of wound patients. The prevention of malnutrition should be a key factor, since the development of certain types of lesions can present a non-apparent but significant loss of protein, resulting in a decrease in the immune and inflammatory response, requiring more time to acquire resistance in the new tissue. Therefore, the aim of this study was to present the benefits of nutritional therapy associated with the use of barbatimao in the wound healing process.

2 MATERIAL AND METHODS

In terms of its objectives, this is an exploratory bibliographical review, which was carried out by searching the Medline, Lilacs, Scielo, Google Scholar and Capes Periodicals databases.

Of the 150 articles and books researched, 76 were selected. For the selection of the sample, the following inclusion criteria were established: national and international studies, in Portuguese and English, which addressed diet therapy and herbal treatment in the tissue healing process, available in full electronically and published between 1986 and 2015. Articles that did not address the chosen topic, scientific articles that were not available in full electronically and outside the 1986-2015 timeframe were excluded.

According to Boccato (2006), bibliographical research seeks to answer a problem (hypothesis) through published theoretical references, checking and discussing the various scientific contributions. This type of research will provide information on what has been researched, how and from what perspective and/or point of view the subject presented in the scientific literature has been dealt with. It is therefore of substantial importance that the researcher carries out a systematic planning of the research process, from the definition of the topic, through the logical construction of the work to the decision on how it will be communicated and disseminated.

3 Results and discussion

3.1 Nutritional Therapy in the Healing Process

Nutritional therapy aims to: offer favorable conditions for establishing the therapeutic plan; guarantee adequate protein and energy supplies to minimize protein catabolism and nitrogen loss, offer energy, recover the activity of the immune system; fluids and nutrients in adequate quantities to maintain vital functions and homeostasis; reduce the risks of exacerbated food intake (MATOS; ROZENFELD; MARTINS, 2008).

Tissue repair comprises three sequential phases: inflammatory, proliferative and maturation, each of which is balanced by growth factors, which are polypeptides that control cell multiplication, growth, differentiation and metabolism (MANDELBAUM; DI SANTIS; MANDELBAUM, 2003).

The inflammatory phase is the phase that follows the injury, lasting four to six days. At the tissue level, there are some changes. In this process, vitamin K is used to synthesize prothrombin and coagulation factors VIII, IX and X. Its function is to minimize blood loss resulting from vessel damage and to create a structure into which fibroblasts will migrate (MAYES; GOTTSCHLICH, 2003).

Phagocytosis takes place in which amino acids are consumed. As a result of the formation of chemotactic factors, neutrophils appear in the lesion to phagocytize bacteria and thus inhibit wound infection. Monocytes differentiate into macrophages and eliminate clots, cell debris, bacteria and necrotic tissue and secrete monokines that will attract repair cells to the wound (MATOS; ROZENFELD; MARTINS, 2008).

The proliferative phase begins on the third day after the injury and lasts for weeks. In this phase, also called the granulation and fibroplasia phase, the main activities observed are:

proliferation of epithelial cells and fibroblasts. In this phase, proteins, vitamin A, zinc, carbohydrates and, indirectly, B vitamins, fats and magnesium are used; collagen synthesis. Amino acids, vitamin C and iron are used for this (MANDELBAUM; DI SANTIS; MANDELBAUM, 2003).

Neovascularization occurs from vessels around the wound site.

These new vessels will enable the supply of energy and oxygen for healing, increasing the wound's resistance to infection. When wounds heal by second intention, the granulation tissue that forms is very important, as it will serve as a vascular bed for the new tissue that will form later (GUENTER et al., 2000).

The maturation or remodeling phase is a process that can last up to two years. During this phase, the collagen stabilizes and the strength of the scar increases (GUENTER et al., 2000). Vitamins are used as co-factors by different enzymes in the healing process. Seriously ill patients may experience a greater loss of vitamins, which can lead to vitamin deficiency and delayed healing. The ideal levels of supplementation for these patients have not yet been defined, and should be taken with care when there is effective data to indicate a deficiency (MAYES; GOTTSCHLICH, 2003).

3.2 Nutrient Relationships in the Healing Process

3.2.1 Carbohydrates

Carbohydrates, specifically glucose, are the main energy source in the development of healing and are important for various cell types, including fibroblasts, leukocytes, endothelial and epithelial cells (ARNOLD; BARBUL, 2006). Carbohydrates play a role in cell propagation, phagocytosis and fibroblast allocation, and are recommended at around 50% to 60% of the energy substrate (MOREIRA JUNIOR, 2006).

During the healing process, there is a condition of hypercatabolism, because on the one hand it is essential to synthesize proteins that are crucial for tissue recovery, and on the other hand it is necessary to boost the immune system. Therefore, carbohydrates are a source of energy for leukocytes and fibroblasts and their deficiency can slow down the healing process.

(DEMLING, 2009).

3.2.2 Proteins and Amino Acids

Protein is essential for maintaining skin integrity. It plays a fundamental role in healing, enabling revascularization, the dissemination of fibroblasts, collagen synthesis and the formation of lymphocytes (MEDEIROS et al., 2009).

In the study by Breslow et al. (1993), it was found that providing too much protein to patients with ulcers (24% of the total amount) contributed to better healing. The protein requirements of an individual with a moderately stressed UPP increase from 1.2 to 1.5 g/kg of weight/day and from 1.5 to 2.0 g/kg/day if the stress is severe (CHEMIN; MURA, 2011).

Proteins play a variety of roles in the body. The role of proteins in the healing process is clear and their deficiency slows down this process in acute and chronic wounds. This is especially clear in UPP and acute burns (SCHOLS; HEYMAN; MEIJER, 2009). During the healing process, in the event of an energy deficiency, protein reserves act as an energy source (COLLINS; KERSHAW; BROCKINGTON, 2005).

Proteins are basic elements of cells and it is understood that protein depletion increases the length of the inflammatory phase; it makes fibroblast proliferation impossible; it minimizes the condensation and deposition of collagen and proteoglycans; represses the tensile strength of the wound, limits the phagocytic efficiency of leukocytes and increases the rate of wound infection; inhibits angiogenesis (SCHOLS; HEYMAN; MEIJER, 2009) and makes it impossible to remodel the wound, i.e. protein deficiency impairs all phases of healing (MACKAY; MILLER, 2003).

Theoretically, the most important activity of proteins in wound patients is tissue and cell growth and repair (COLLINS; KERSHAW; BROCKINGTON, 2005). Guenter et al. (2000) show that the majority of patients who have recently been hospitalized with severe pressure ulcers are malnourished. Breslow et al. (2003) concluded that hyperprotein diets can improve the healing process in malnourished patients with wounds.

Van Anholt et al. (2010) found that nutritional protein supplementation helps to reduce the intensity of pressure ulcers in malnourished patients, reducing treatment costs.

The articles consulted point to the efficacy of proteins in the healing process, with a consensus among the authors on their use in malnourished and nourished patients and on the fact that a large number of inpatients have protein deficiencies.

3.2.3 Arginine

Arginine is an essential amino acid and is low in the body in situations of metabolic stress

(DEMLING, 2009). Arginine is closely related to wound healing as it is the predecessor of proline, developing the tensile strength of the wound (SCHOLS; HEYMAN; MEIJER, 2009). Table (1) lists the most current studies on arginine in the healing process, summarizing the agreement on the positive factors of using arginine in the diet in the healing process, as well as the contribution of this amino acid to the immune system.

Table 1. Studies on the role of arginine in the healing process.

Title	Authors/ Year	Sample	Results
Nutritional therapy in burns: a review	Silva et al. (2012).	Burn patients	Glutamine, arginine, omega 3 and vitamins A, C, E, zinc and selenium are important in the healing process and act on the immune system.
The role of arginine and glutamine in immunomodulation in burn patients: a literature review	Sousa et al. (2015).	Burn patients	The administration of arginine and glutamine is beneficial and appears to be an essential alternative intervention in the treatment of metabolic alterations involved in the pathophysiology of burns.

In some studies, arginine supplementation has been shown to improve protein metabolism, helping to reduce muscle loss and collagen synthesis, which supports the healing process (BAUER; ISENRING; WATERHOUSE, 2013; CEREDA et al., 2015).

Van Anholt et al. (2010) found in their study that nutritional supplementation of arginine helps to reduce the intensity of UPP in malnourished patients, reducing treatment costs.

3.2.4 Glutamine

Glutamine is the most numerous amino acid in the body. This amino acid is considered conditionally essential, since under circumstances of metabolic stress, its plasma accumulation decreases rapidly (DEMLING, 2009). In the course of this, glutamine is used in gluconeogenesis as the primary source of energy (MACKAY; MILLER, 2003), in order for cells to divide rapidly. It is vital in inciting the inflammatory response, as it stimulates lymphocyte formation (energy substrate for lymphocytes). It also has an antioxidant action, defending the body against the toxic effects of ammonia (MOLNAR, 2007). It also has anabolic and anticatabolic properties, acting as a precursor in the synthesis of purines, pyrimidines and phospholipids, and contributes to the integrity of the intestine (DEMLING, 2009).

Glutamine has several properties that demonstrate its important function in the normal and pathophysiological state. Of the total *pool of* intracellular free amino acids, glutamine accounts for approximately 60% (MOSKOVITZ, 1994).

Blass et al. (2013) showed that deprivation of this amino acid can lead to an increase in the difficulty of healing. Laboratory and clinical data show that glutamine is considered an essential amino acid during certain conditions of catabolic stress (LEE et al., 2005; LIN et al., 2005; HUCKLEBERRY, 2004).

Despite glutamine's obvious contribution to some physiological processes, there are few publications validating glutamine in the healing process, so further research into the role of this amino acid is suggested.

3.2.5 Lipids

Lipids are involved in cell membrane synthesis, prostaglandin formation, cell metabolism and the development of vascular inflammation (TERR et al., 2004).

It is understood that lipids are an integral part of cell membranes and also function as signaling molecules; sources of substrate for the various functions of their by-products, especially the components of free fatty acids, are sources of cellular energy. Lipids are part of the wound process, inflammation, proliferation and play a fundamental role in tissue production and wound remodulation (DEMLING, 2009).

White adipose tissue is a source of pro-inflammatory fat and is one of the essential regulators of inflammation and wound healing (DEMLING, 2009). A lack of essential fatty acids, such as linoleic acid (n-6) and arachidonic acid (AA), weakens wound healing (MAYES; GOTTSCHILCH, 2003) because they are precursors or components of phospholipids and prostaglandins, which are essential, in that order, in the structure of the cell membrane and in the metabolic, inflammatory and vascular functions of the cell (ARNOLD; BARBUL, 2006).

The cytokines provided by omega-3 are prostaglandins-3 and thromboxanes-3, which have the clear purpose of reducing platelet aggregation, reducing pre-inflammatory capacity and immunomodulation in the inflammatory response. The recommendation for omega-3 is 0.1 to 0.2 g of fish oil/kg/day (ROSINA; COSTA, 2010).

Lipids are classified as essential and non-essential. Iinoleic acid and linolenic acid are essential in humans. With Iinoleic acid, the body synthesizes arachidonic acid and Iinoleic acid. Iinoleic acid plays a significant role in preserving the epidermal water barrier (DINIZ, 2013).

Linolenic acid is a precursor of biological membrane elements and prostaglandin. In addition, unsaturated lipids are important for transporting lipids in the blood, which in turn are crucial for producing the greatest amount of energy and transporting fat-soluble vitamins (vitamins A, D, E and K) (DINIZ, 2013).

Najmi et al. (2015) observed that olive oil has antioxidant properties, including hydrocarbons, polyphenols and triterpenoids, consequently generating a protective anti-inflammatory effect, favoring the healing process. However, nutritional support with more than 15% of calories coming from lipids impairs its function in the immune system.

In a study of 23 adult burn patients in serious condition (>25% CWS), they were occasionally assigned to three types of nutritional assistance, differing in the portion of energy derived from lipid and the presence or absence of fish oil. Group I (control), 35% lipid, group II, 15% lipid, group III, 15% lipid with 50% fish oil. Nutritional assistance was both parenteral and enteral and introduced within 24 hours of hospitalization. This study showed that, in burns, the serum accumulation of somatomedins (IGF-I) is vulnerable to the type of lipid in the nutritional support. The addition of fish oil to the diet enabled IGF-I levels in serum to be re-established more quickly (ABRIBAT et al., 2000).

In another study, Najmi et al. (2015) demonstrated that an oral diet supplied with olive oil in patients with wounds can speed up the wound healing process and shorten the patient's hospitalization period. While Hatanaka (2007) suggests that a nutritional deficiency of fatty acids slows down the healing process.

The studies presented show that lipids have an excellent effect on the healing process, reducing hospitalization time and the suffering of individuals with various wounds.

3.2.6 Ascorbic Acid (Vitamin C)

Vitamin C is a water-soluble vitamin that is essential for healing and its deficiency slows down this process (MOREIRA JÙNIOR, 2006). This vitamin is essential for the hydroxylation of proline and lysine in the synthesis of collagen (DONER; POSTHAUER; THOMAS, 2009). It increases phagocytosis and can increase the activation of leukocytes and macrophages in the wound. In addition to its efficient antioxidant activities, it intervenes in the construction of abnormal collagen fibers (MACKAY; MILLER, 2003).

It is understood that its deficiency minimizes the chemotaxis of neutrophils and monocytes (ARNOLD; BARBUL, 2006), also decreases the tensile strength of fibrous tissues, increases capillary fragility (MOREIRA JÙNIOR, 2006), changes in the intracellular matrix, manifested by skin lesions, weak endothelial cell junctions, hinders local antibacterial defense and increases the viability of recently epithelialized wounds (MACKAY; MILLER, 2003).

Table (2) shows the most current studies on the action of ascorbic acid (Vitamin C) in the healing process.

Table 2. Studies on the role of ascorbic acid in the healing process.

Title	Authors/ Year	Sample	Results
Action of ascorbic acid on the healing process of cutaneous wounds in malnourished rats	Manzoli (2013).	ascorbic acid in 22 malnourished male rats. Induced incision.	Ascorbic acid was effective in healing malnourished and nourished rats.
Evaluation of the use of ascorbic acid supplementation in the healing of cutaneous wounds in diabetic rats	Pereira et al. (2012)	Ascorbic acid in 32 diabetic male rats. Incision induced.	Ascorbic acid was effective in the healing process of diabetic and non-diabetic rats.

Vitamin C boosts resistance to infections, improves phagocytosis and stimulates leukocytes and macrophages in the affected area (ARAÙJO; SANTOS, 2009).

Reddy, Gill and Rochon (2006) found that low concentrations of vitamin C seem to be associated with the appearance of ulcers in elderly people with femoral fractures. However, the effects of vitamin C supplementation on the development of wounds are only seen in conditions of severe depletion. Supplementation with high doses of vitamin C has not been shown to stimulate the healing of PUs.

Several studies have shown that vitamin C supplementation helps to promote healing of pressure ulcers (ARMSTRONG et al., 2014; BLASS et al., 2013; CEREDA et al., 2015; VAN ANHOLT et al., 2010).

In view of the data collected, it can be said that ascorbic acid deficiency in individuals with UPP can cause damage to the healing process, as well as accelerating the healing process when supplemented.

3.2.7 Zinc

Zinc is found in small amounts in the body (SCHOLS; HEYMAN; MEIJER, 2009). The body retains between 2 and 3g, with 1/5 in the bone, 1/2 in the liver and the rest in the muscle (MOLNAR, 2007). Zinc is the most significant of the trace elements in the healing process, playing a considerable role in all phases of healing. However, it plays a greater role in the final stages of tissue repair and regeneration than during the initial infamous phase (GRAY, 2003). A decrease in zinc levels in the body can lead to problems such as chronic wounds and delayed healing (BERGER et al., 2007).

According to Moraes et al. (2000), in a study of 53 diabetic rats, insulin treatment and dietary supplementation of zinc and chromium favored the healing of skin wounds.

Zinc works by stimulating the process of cell mitosis and the dissemination of fibroblasts, thus improving the healing of UPP, as well as having a phagocytic and immune function and favoring taste and appetite (CHEMIN; MURA, 2011).

After the injury, the body redistributes zinc, increasing the levels in the wound and minimizing them in the skin. Due to hypermetabolism, there is an increased loss of zinc in the urine. Its deficiency has adverse consequences for wound healing as it is related to a reduction in the rate of epithelialization, a decrease in tensile strength, a decrease in fibroblast function and a decrease in cellular and humoral immune function, increasing the wound's susceptibility to infection (DEMLING, 2009).

Deficiency of these elements slows down the healing process, leading to a loss of tensile strength in the scar and a reduction in the inflammatory response. The recommended daily dose of zinc for patients with severe wounds in adults is 220 mg (SORIANO et al., 2004).

In the study carried out by the above-mentioned author with 39 patients with grade III and IV pressure ulcers, the effectiveness of an oral supplement with a high protein content enriched with arginine, vitamin C and zinc was evaluated. There was a significant reduction in the area of the ulcers and restoration of the lesions after three weeks. Thus, the findings of the present studies indicate that zinc helps to reduce wounds, contributing to the individual's improvement.

3.2.8 Vitamin A

Vitamin A is a fat-soluble vitamin deposited in the liver, which is essential for bone and epithelial growth, cell differentiation and the work of the immune system (GRAY, 2003).

Vitamin A also reverses the anti-inflammatory effects of corticosteroids on healing, as it induces the inflammatory response by promoting the influx of monocytes and macrophages, developing and triggering the immune response at the site (ARNOLD; BARBUL, 2006).

Vitamin A (retinol) is necessary for the preservation of normal epidermis and for the synthesis of glycoproteins and proteoglycans. It has the function of increasing the metabolism of epithelial cells and their division. It acts strongly on the immune system. Its deficiency slows down the re-epithelialization of wounds, the synthesis of collagen and increases sensitivity to infections (CHEMIN; MURA, 2011).

Vitamin A acts in the processing of collagen synthesis and consolidation and in epithelialization, contributes to the health of the epidermis, enhances tensile strength and resistance to infection (WAITZBERG; RASLAN; RAVACCI, 2009).

Animal studies have shown that vitamin A supplementation can prevent scar damage in the presence of tumors and after radiation. Regarding doses, there is no general consensus, however, some authors suggest supplementation when there is evidence of deficiency and for a short period of time (BOTTONI et al., 2011).

The articles found show that vitamin A has beneficial effects on accelerating wound healing and also improves the immune system.

3.2.9 B-complex vitamins

The B vitamins (B1, B2, B3, biotin, B5, B6, B9 and B12) are still going through the process of defining their roles in the various phases of wound healing. However, it is clear that the vitamins in this complex have characteristic metabolic attributes and that they are related to each other, with the aim of ensuring that energy metabolism and tissue synthesis in the wound take place properly (ARNOLD; BARBUL, 2006).

They play a crucial role in the proliferation and remodeling phases, where they are involved in the synthesis of interconnections in the collagen molecule and in the formation of new tissues and blood vessels. During the final phase of healing, myofibroblasts depend on B vitamins for wound reduction (MOLNAR, 2007).

Molnar (2007) also found in his study that several studies confirm that B vitamins are associated with coenzymes that work at the beginning of the inflammatory phase and during the removal of bacteria and necrotic tissue.

Neiva et al. (2005) found in their study that vitamin B supplementation in patients with UPP improved healing compared to the placebo group.

3.3 Herbal medicines

Over the last few decades, researchers have sought to use unconventional materials and methods to treat wounds. Currently, the demand for herbal medicines has increased dramatically, and the use of these products to treat various ailments has become increasingly notorious. At the same time, the development of new pharmaceutical forms and control techniques guarantees quality for health professionals and the safety of prescribing herbal medicines that the population has used for a long time (BERGER et al., 2003).

The scientific literature shows the use of herbal medicines with various therapeutic indications, including for treating wounds, some of which are well-established and belong to the Brazilian pharmacopoeia (MARTINS et al., 2003).

3.3.1 Barbatimào (*Stryphnodendron adstringens* (Mart.) Coville)

A widely used phytotherapeutic is Barbatimao, popularly known as barbatimao, barba-de-timao, barbatimao-verdade, barca-da-mocidade, barca-da- virginity, charaozinho-roxo, iba-timò, uabatimò and verna. A low-growing plant from the *Fabaceae* family, subfamily *Mimosoidae*. It has small palmate leaves with oval leaflets, small reddish or whitish flowers gathered in cylindrical spikes, and fruit in the form of thick, scaly pods enclosing seeds similar to beans (CORRÊA; BATISTA; QUINTAS, 2011).

It adapts best to dry, well-drained soils and full sunlight. In addition to its therapeutic action, it is widely used for dyeing leather and making paints. Its chemical composition includes acids (ellagic, gallic), flavonoids, tannins, alkaloids, terpenes, stilbenes, steroids, trypsin and protease inhibitors, sugars and mucilage. The part used is the bark (CORRÊA; BATISTA; QUINTAS, 2011).

The barbatimao contains 20% tannin in its bark, an active ingredient that gives it an astringent action, which makes it suitable for use as a healing agent. It has also been reported that the aqueous extract of *Stryphnodendron adstringens* (Mart.) Coville has anti-inflammatory, analgesic and gastric mucosa protective properties (BEZERRA et al., 2002; REBECCA et al., 2002).

The antinociceptive activity of the crude extract of barbatimao has also been studied, and the results suggest that the extract has an antinociceptive effect through peripheral mechanisms (MELO et al., 2007). Other activities have also been described in the literature for this species, such as trypanocidal (HERZOG- SOARES et al., 2002) and anti-inflammatory (FALCÂO et al., 2005).

Souza et al. (2007) analyzed the antiseptic and antimicrobial activity of the dry extract of Barbatimao against two gram-positive and one gram-negative bacteria. The results were positive for *Staphylococcus aureus*, *Staphylococcus epidermidis and Escherichia coli*, as well as antiseptic activity.

3.3.2 Formulations

There are various formulations for its use, some of the most widespread are: tinctures, ointments, soaps.

Tinctures are solutions manipulated from the extraction of plants with an alcoholic or hydroalcoholic solution at room temperature. Tinctures can be a final product when used directly by the patient (for example, tinctures of Calendula, Arnica, Barbatimao, etc.) or a raw material when incorporated into formulations for typical use (ointments, creams and gels) or internal use (syrups) (CORRÊA; BATISTA; QUINTAS, 2011).

Medicinal soaps are used for personal hygiene, but they also serve as a vehicle for medicinal substances. The amount of active ingredients that remain on the body is small due to the rinsing process. It is easy to use and can be distributed quickly throughout the body (CORRÊA; BATISTA; QUINTAS, 2011).

4 CONCLUSIONS

It is important to carry out a nutritional assessment in order to recognize possible malnutrition or vitamin and mineral deficiencies early on, thus generating more effective interventions to speed up the healing process. In some cases, setbacks in healing are linked to low-calorie, low-protein diets and micronutrient and mineral deficiencies. The nutrients involved in the healing process are proteins (arginine and glutamine), lipids, carbohydrates, vitamins A, B, C, D and E and zinc.

The role of nutrients in the wound healing process is to slow down the progression of healing, provide energy for the process, maintain adequate hydration and achieve excellent results. It is worth emphasizing that nutritional care is essential because the longer the healing time, the greater the value of health care for wound patients. Adequate nutritional status provides effective healing with excellent results for the patient.

The palliative use of *Stryphnodendron adstringens* (Mart.) Coville contributes to improving the wound healing process, as has been shown in various studies, due to the components found in Barbatimao with healing, anti-inflammatory, hemostatic, antiseptic, anti-diarrheal, anti-edematogenic, antinociceptive and antimicrobial activities. However, it is necessary to buy it from certified and reliable sources, as there can be a wide variation in quality and safety.

Despite the importance of the studies found on the subject, there is a need for more specific research on diet therapy applied to wound healing, especially with regard to nutrients: carbohydrates, vitamin A, vitamin E and B vitamins. Few studies were found for debate. It is also worth highlighting the scarcity of recent studies on the barbatimao *Stryphnodendron adstringens* (Mart.) Coville, making more relevant research into its therapeutic properties necessary.

REFERENCES

ABRIBAT, T. et al. Decreased serum insulin-like growth factor I in burn patients: relationship with serum insulin-like growth factor binding protein-3 proteolysis and the influence of lipid composition in nutritional support. **Critical Care Medicine**, v. 28, n.7, p. 2366-72, 2000.

ARAÙJO, A. R.; SANTOS, Z. A. Dietotherapy in the Prevention and Treatment of Pressure Ulcers. **Nutriçâo em Pauta**, v. 17, n. 98, p. 44-48, 2009.

ARNOLD, M.; BARBUL, A. Nutrition and wound healing. **Plastic and Reconstructive Surgery,** v. 117, n. 7, p. 42-58, 2006.

BAUER, J. D.; ISENRING, E.; WATERHOUSE, M. The effectiveness of a specialized oral nutrition supplement on outcomes in patients with chronic wounds: A pragmatic randomized study. **Journal of Human Nutrition and Dietetics**, v. 26, n. 5, p. 452-458, 2013.

BERGER, M. M. et al. Trace element supplementation after major burns modulates antioxidant statusand clinical course by way of increased tissue trace element concentrations. **American Journal of Clinical Nutrition**, v. 85, n. 5, p. 1293-300, 2007.

BEZERRA, J. C. B. et al. Molluscicidal activity against Biomphalaria glabrata of Brazilian Cerrado medicinal plants. **Fitoterapia**, v.73, p.428-430, 2002.

BLASS, S. C. et al. Extracellular micronutrient levels and pro-/antioxidant status in trauma patients with wound healing disorders: results of a cross-sectional study.

Nutrition Journal, v. 12, n. 1, p. 157, 2013.

BOCCATO, V. R. C. Metodologia da pesquisa bibliogràfica na área odontológica e o artigo cientifico como forma de comunicaçao. **Revista de Odontologia da Univiversidade de Cidade Sâo Paulo**, v. 18, n. 3, p. 265-274, 2006.

BOTTONI, A. et al. Role of Nutrition in Healing. **Revista Ciências em Saùde**, v. 1, n. 1, p. 1-5, 2011.

BRESLOW, R. A. et al. The importance of dietary protein in realing pressure ulcer. **Journal of the American Geriatrics Society**, v. 41, n. 4, p. 357-62, 1993.

CEREDA, E. et al. A Nutritional Formula Enriched With Arginine, Zinc, and Antioxidants for the Healing of Pressure Ulcers. **Annals of Internal Medicine**, v. 162, n. 3, p. 167-74, 2015.

CHEMIN, S. M. S. S.; MURA, J. D. P. **Treatise on Food, Nutrition and Diet Therapy**. Sao Paulo: Roca, 2011.

COLLINS, C. E.; KERSHAW, J.; BROCKINGTON, S. Effect of nutritional supplements on wound healing in home-nursed elderly: a randomized trial.

Nutrition, v. 21, n. 2, p.147-55, 2005.

CORRÊA, A. D.; BATISTA, R. S.; QUINTAS, L. E. M. **Plantas Medicinais: do cultivo à terapèutica.** 8ª ed., Rio de Janeiro, Editora Petrópolis, 2011.

DEALEY, C. **Wound care: a guide for nurses.** 3rd ed. Sao Paulo: Atheneu , 2008.

DEMLING, R. H. Nutrition, anabolism, and the wound healing process: anoverview. **Eplasty,** v. 9, p. 9, 2009.

DINIZ, A. G. **Relevance of nutrition in the wound healing process.**

Federal University of Minas Gerais. Faculty of Medicine. Collective Health Education Center. Lagoa Santa, 2013.

DORNER, B.; POSTHAUER, M. E.; THOMAS, D. The Role of Nutrition in Pressure Ulcer Prevention and Treatment: National Pressure Ulcer Advisory Panel White Paper. **Advances in Skin & Wound Care**, v. 22, n. 5, p. 212-21, 2009.

FALCÂO, H. S. et al. Review of the plants with anti-infl ammatory activity studied in Brazil. **Revista Brasileira de Farmacognosia**, v.15, p. 381-391, 2005.

GRAY, M. Does oral supplementation with vitamins A or E promote healing of chronic wounds? **Journal of Wound Ostomy & Continence Nursing**, v. 30, n. 6, p. 290-4, 2003.

GUENTER, P. et al. Survey of nutritional status in newly hospitalized patients with stage III or stage IV pressure ulcers. **Advances in Skin & Wound Care**, v. 13, p.164-8, 2000.

HATANAKA, E. Fatty acids and healing: a review. **Revista Brasileira de Farmàcia**, v. 88, n. 2, p. 53-58, 2007.

HERZOG-SOARES, J. D. et al. In vivo trypanocidal activity of *Stryphnodendron adstringens* (barbatimao verdadeiro) and *Caryocar brasiliensis* (pequi). **Revista Brasileira de Farmacognosia**, v.12, n.1, p. 1-2, 2002.

HUCKLEBERRY, Y. Nutritional support and the surgical patient. **American Journal of Health-System Pharmacy**, v. 61, p. 671-684, 2004.

LEE, C. H. et al. Effects of glutamine-containing total parenteral nutrition on phagocytic activity and anabolic hormone response in rats undergoing gastrectomy.

World Journal of Gastroenterology, v. 11, n. 6, p. 817-822, 2005.

LIN, M. T. et al. Glutamine-supplemented total parenteral nutrition attenuates plasma interleukin-6 in surgical patients with lower disease severity. **World Journal of Gastroenterology**, v. 11, n. 39, p. 6197-6201, 2005.

MACKAY, D.; MILLER, A. L. Nutritional Support for Wound Healing.

Alternative Medicine Review, v. 8, n. 4, p. 359-377, 2003.

MANDELBAUM, S. H.; DI SANTIS, E. P.; MANDELBAUM, M. H. S.

Healing: Current concepts and auxiliary resources - Part I. **Anais Brasileiros de Dermatologia**, v. 78, n. 4, p. 393-420, 2003.

MANZOLI, L. M. F. **Action of ascorbic acid on the healing of cutaneous wounds in malnourished rats.** Dissertation (Master's Degree in Animal Science) - Universidade do Oeste Paulista - Unoeste, Presidente Prudente, SP, 2013.

MARTINS, P. S. et al. Comparison of typical herbal medicines in equine skin healing. **Archives of Veterinary Science**, v.8, p.1-7, 2003.

MATOS, G. C.; ROZENFELD, S.; MARTINS, M. Human albumin prescribed for cases of malnutrition in hospitals in Rio de Janeiro. **Revista da Associaçâo Médica Brasileira**, v. 54, n. 3, p. 220-4, 2008.

MAYES, T.; GOTTSCHLICH, M. M. Burns and wound healing. In: MATARESE, L. E.; GOTTSCHLICH, M. M. **Conteporary Nutrition Support Practice**. St. Louis, Mo.

Luis: Saunders, p. 595-615, 2003.

MEDEIROS, N. I et al. Effects of enteral nutritional therapy in burn patients treated at a public hospital in Joinville/SC. **Revista Brasileira de Queimaduras**, v. 8, n. 3, p. 97-100, 2009.

MELO, J. O. et al. Effect of Stryphnodendron adstringens (barbatimao) bark on animal models of nociception. **Revista Brasileira de Ciências Farmacêuticas**, v. 43, n. 3, p. 465-469, 2007.

MOLNAR, J. A. **Nutrition and wound healing**. Boca Raton, Fla.; London: CRC, 360p, 2007.

MORAES, S. P. et al. Zinc and chromium in wound healing in normal and diabetic rats. **Revista do Colégio Brasileiro de Cirurgioes**, v. 27, n. 6, p. 394-399, 2000.

MOREIRA JÙNIOR, J.C. Malnutrition and Wound Healing. In:

WAITZBERG, D. L. **Oral, Enteral and Parenteral Nutrition in Clinical Practice.**

3ªed, v. 1, Sao Paulo: Atheneu, p. 411-421, 2006.

MOSKOVITZ, B. et al. Glutamine metabolism and utilization: relevance to major problems in health care. **Pharmacological Research**, v. 30, n. 1, p. 61-71, 1994.

NAJMI, M. et al. Effect of oral olive oil on healing of 10-20% total body surface area burn wounds in hospitalized patients. **Burns**, v. 41, n. 3, p. 493-6, 2015.

NEIVA, R. F. et al. Effects of vitamin-B complex supplementation on periodontal wound healing. **Journal of Periodontology**, v. 76, p. 1084-1091, 2005.

ORGILL, D.; DEMLING, R. H. Current concepts and approaches to wound healing. **Critical Care Medicine**, v. 16, n. 9, p. 899-908, 1988.

PEREIRA, S. C. L. et al. Evaluation of the use of ascorbic acid supplementation in the healing of cutaneous wounds in diabetic rats. **Revista do Médico Residente**, v. 14, n. 4, p. 236-247,

2012.

SCHOLS, J. M.; HEYMAN, H.; MEIJER, E. P. Nutritional support in the treatment and prevention of pressure ulcers: An overview of studies with an arginine enriched Oral Nutritional Supplement. **Journal of Tissue Viability**, v. 18, n. 3, p. 72-9, 2009.

SILVA, A. P. A. et al. Nutritional therapy in burns: a review. **Revista Brasileira de Queimaduras**, v. 11, n. 3, p. 135-41, 2012.

SORIANO, F. L. et al. The effectiveness of oral nutritional supplementation in the healing of pressure ulcers. **Journal of Wound Care**, v.13, n. 8, p. 319-22, 2004.

SOUSA, A. E. S. et al. The role of arginine and glutamine in immunomodulation in burn patients - literature review. **Revista Brasileira de Queimaduras**, v. 14, n. 4, p. 295-9, 2015.

SOUZA, T. M. et al. Evaluation of the antiseptic activity of a dry extract of *Stryphnodendron adstringens* (Mart.) Coville and a cosmetic preparation containing this extract. **Brazilian Journal of Pharmacognosy**, v. 17, p. 71-75, 2007.

REBECCA, M.A. et al. Toxicological studies on *Stryphnodendron adstringens*.

Journal of Ethnopharmacol., v.83, p.101-104, 2002.

REDDY, M.; GILL, S. S.; ROCHON, P. A. Preventing pressure ulcers: a systematic review. **JAMA**, v. 296, n. 8, p. 974-84, 2006.

ROSINA, K.T.C.; COSTA, C.L. Use of immunomodulatory nutritional therapy in polytraumatized patients: a literature review. **Ceres**, v. 5, n. 2, p. 27-36, 2010.

TERR, A. I. et al. **Medical Immunology**. Editora Guanabara-Koogan, 10ª edition, 2004.

VAN ANHOLT, R. D. et al. Specific nutritional support accelerates pressure ulcer healing and reduces wound care intensity in non-malnourished patients. **Nutrition**, v. 26, n. 9, p. 867-872, 2010.

WAITZBERG, D.L.; RASLAN, M.; RAVACCI, G.R. Malnutrition: Prevalence and Metabolism. In: WAITZBERG, D.L. **Oral, Enteral and Parenteral Nutrition in Clinical Practice**. 4th ed., v.1, Sâo Paulo: Atheneu, p. 535-5, 2009.

CHAPTER 4

PHYTOTHERAPY AND ITS IMPORTANCE IN NATURAL AND NUTRITIONAL THERAPY: A REVIEW

Lusimere Almeida de Oliveira[1]

Maria das Graças Silva[2]

1. Postgraduate student in Clinical Nutrition: Metabolism, Practice and Nutritional Therapy at the Cândido Mendes University (UCAM-RJ);

2. Master's Degree in Natural and Synthetic Bioactive Products, Federal University of Paraiba.

ABSTRACT: Phytotherapy is defined as the science that studies the use of products of plant origin for therapeutic purposes to prevent, mitigate or cure a pathological condition. The aim of this study was therefore to analyze the importance of phytotherapy used as a natural and nutritional therapy. This is a bibliographic study, through a literature review of national and international journals collected from Medline, Lilacs and Scielo databases, as well as the use of monographs, dissertations and theses from the various health areas related to the topic. Phytotherapy is an ancient, simple and natural form of treatment that cures or prevents diseases through plant preparations. It is part of the practice of folk medicine, based on the same principle as allopathic medicine through active ingredients, requiring care. Given this context, it can be concluded that phytotherapy is an area of extreme importance both as a natural therapy and as a nutritional therapy. As a natural therapy, it stands out for being a simple and natural treatment, more accessible, low cost and with low side effects, as it is an effective form of primary health care, complementing the drug treatment usually used by the poor. Nutritional therapy through phytotherapy has been gaining ground in relation to foods and their functional properties, preventing diseases and providing a better quality of life for the population. According to CFN Resolution No. 556 of April 11, 2015, the practice of phytotherapy is regulated for nutritionists to complement dietary prescriptions.

Keywords: Medicinal plants. Natural Therapy. Nutritional Therapy. Phytotherapy.

1 INTRODUCTION

Phytotherapy is defined as the science that studies the use of products of plant origin for therapeutic purposes to prevent, mitigate or cure a pathological condition. In this context, phytotherapy encompasses medicinal plants, extracts and herbal medicines

(VANACLOCHA; FOLCARA, 2003).

The World Health Organization (WHO) recognizes herbal medicine as a science that has been studied, perfected and applied over the years, so it can no longer be considered just knowledge passed down from parents to children (SCHULZ; HANSEL; TYLER, 2002).

In Brazil, the emergence of folk medicine with the use of plants is characterized by the culture of the Indians, blacks and Europeans (FERREIRA et al., 2014).

Phytotherapy is used in several countries, including Egypt, where the Egyptians made a great contribution by using plants not only to cure diseases, but also to embalm bodies and for religious rituals in which they used plants with various properties, including aromatic, antiseptic and cosmetic, as well as cultivating purgative, diuretic and vermifuge plants (CORDEIRO; NUNES; ALMEIDA, 1996; BRAGANÇA, 1996).

Around 3,000 years BC in China, there are reports of cures using folk medicine, and it is considered to be the cradle of the use of medicinal plants. In addition, the Chinese, Egyptians, Hindus and Greeks classified medicinal plants according to their shape, taste and aroma, including links with the stars and, of course, their magical attributes (ARAÙJO, 2007).

In the Middle Ages, there was an interest in the material world, which came to be seen as the center of the universe due to the changes that favored capitalist production, which maintained man's active labor force, guaranteeing the production of factories and not valuing the healing activities of plants (ALVIN et al., 2006).

Phytotherapy has been the fastest growing integrative medicine over the years. In the world drug market, the sale of phytochemicals is worth around 15 billion dollars. The most important factor for this growth is the evolution of scientific studies, in particular the discovery of the efficacy of medicinal plants, especially those used by the population for therapeutic purposes, through chemical and pharmacological studies (CECHINEL-FILHO; YUNES, 1998).

The use of popular knowledge as a basis for scientific research into medicinal plants has gained impact in recent years and has led many health professionals to investigate ways of introducing species into phytotherapy programs in the primary health care network (TOMAZZONI; NEGRELLE; CENTA, 2006).

Therefore, the aim of this work was to analyze the importance of phytotherapy used as a natural and nutritional therapy, as well as to classify the types of therapeutic uses, to present plants as a therapy for disease prevention and to indicate some foods that are important in nutritional therapy.

2 MATERIAL AND METHODS

This is a bibliographical study, using searches in national and international journals in the Medline, Lilacs and Scielo databases, as well as monographs, dissertations and theses from the various health areas related to the topic. Original and review articles, available in full electronically, were used. The following descriptors were used: phytotherapy, therapeutic uses of phytotherapy.

3 RESULTS AND DISCUSSION

Recently, interest in natural therapies has grown significantly. This growth is due to the high cost of industrialized medicines, the side effects they cause, the ease with which medicinal plants can be obtained and, above all, the false idea that products from nature do no harm. These reasons have led to a gradual increase in the consumption of herbal drugs and phytotherapeutic medicines (SIMÔES; SCHENKEL, 2011).

In order to use plants as medicines, ancient peoples used their own experiences and observed the use of plants by animals. Parts of the plant such as the root, stem and leaf can provide active substances that will be used to obtain a medicine (OLIVEIRA; SIMÔES; SASSI, 2006; ROSA; BARCELOS; BAMPI, 2012). In Northeastern culture, medicinal plants are commonly used to prepare home remedies to treat various ailments. These include: lemon balm (*Lippia alba mill*); lemongrass (*Cymbopogon citratus SlapJ.);* rosemary (*Rosmarinus officinalis* L.); green tea (*Camelia sinensis* L.) and chamomile (*Matricaria chamomilla* L.).

According to the literature, lemon balm (*Lippia alba mill)* has proven calming and mild antispasmodic actions, as well as analgesic activity. It is widely used as an infusion of fresh leaves. In cases of minor uterine and intestinal colic and in nervous, restless and insomniac states (sedative action), it can be consumed at will as it has very low toxicity (PINTO; AMOROZO; FURLAN, 2006; MATOS, 2002). Contraindications: pregnant women who are allergic to plants from the *verbenaceae* family, allergy sufferers in general, patients with heart, kidney and liver problems and other patients with chronic illnesses. Dosage for internal use: 0.5 to 2% infusion of the leaves, 3 cups a day after meals (DINIZ, 2006).

Lemongrass (*Cymbopogon citratus Stapf)* has a calming and mild antispasmodic effect. The infusion, freshly prepared from fresh or dried leaves, is useful for relieving small bouts of intestinal and uterine colic, as well as nervousness and restlessness, and has a diuretic action (SINGI et al., 2005). Contraindications: pregnant women, people allergic to the poaceae plant family, allergy sufferers in general, patients with heart, kidney and liver disease and other patients with other chronic illnesses. It should not be combined with drugs that depress the central nervous system (CNS). Dosage: 5 to 6 g of the leaf, preferably dried, or 1 to 3 g of the dried leaves to 1 cup of boiling water and simmer for 10 minutes (DINIZ, 2006).

Rosemary (*Rosmarinus officinalis* L.) is one of the best known medicinal plants since ancient times, thanks to its medicinal, edible and flavoring properties. In ancient Egypt, it was used in formulations for mummification and was very common in monasteries. In ancient Rome, it was used to purify sacred tombs. It can be used as: antibiotic, anti-inflammatory, digestive (hepatoprotective, choleretic), antispasmodic, antioxidant, stimulant, reduces capillary permeability, diuretic, expectorant, antiparasitic, rubefacient (increases local circulation) for topical use. In particular, rosemary is considered to be a plant with marked therapeutic effects and its therapeutic use should be carefully monitored and discontinued immediately if there are undesirable effects (LIMA; LOPPES, 2008). Contraindications: pregnant women who are allergic to plants from the *lamiaceae* family, allergy sufferers in general, cardiac, renal and hepatopathic patients and other patients with chronic illnesses. Dosage: the infusion of the leaves should be used to treat wounds or skin burns immediately after preparation with 10 to 12 leaves in 1 cup of hot water (MATOS, 2002). The tincture used for topical use is prepared with 10 g of the leaves dried in the shade or 20 mg of the fresh leaves in 30 ml of water and 70 ml of water, respectively (MATOS, 2002).

Green tea (*Camelia sinensis* L.) is a diuretic and tonic-stimulating drink, with a milder effect than coffee, but a longer one; it reduces the accumulation of fat in the liver and arteries, lowering blood fat levels (especially cholesterol); has an antioxidant role, acting as a preventative in cardiovascular and oncological diseases (tumors in general); antiviral; inhibits platelet aggregation; reduces muscle pain after physical exertion; also acts as a digestive and anti-acid (ALONSO, 1998).

Chamomile (*Matricaria chamomilla* L.) is used as a calming, digestive, intestinal gas and colic fighter, relaxant, fever, anti-inflammatory, analgesic, antispasmodic, healing, as well as for allergies (MARTINAZZO; MARTINS, 2004). It is contraindicated for pregnant women due to its smooth muscle relaxing activity and for patients with hypersensitivity (ARRUDA et al., 2013) or allergy to plants of the *asteraceae* family. Oral Dosage: administer 150 ml of the infusion (5-10 min after preparation), 3-4 times between meals (over 12 years old) (BRASIL, 2011); administer 1-4 ml of the fluid extract for adults (3 times a day) or 0.6-2 ml in a single dose (children over 3 years old). Do not use in children under 3 years of age (D'IPPOLITO; ROCHA; SILVA, 2005). Mouthwash and/or gargle: administer the infusion (5-10 minutes after preparation), 3 times a day. Topical use: compresses using the infusion prepared with 30-100g of plant drug in 1000 ml of water (WHO, 1999). Infusion: 6-9 g in 150 mL or 30-100 g in 1000mL (WHO, 1999; BRASIL, 2011). Time of use of chamomile: No data was found in the literature on the maximum time of use. The length of use depends on the therapeutic indication and the evolution of the condition monitored by the prescribing professional.

The grape (*Vitis vinifera* L.) is a climbing plant with bushy tendrils. Its leaves are petiolate alternate, cordate, with five toothed sinuate lobes, glabrous on the upper side and tomentose on the underside. The flowers are small and greenish-white, arranged in racemes (SCHLEIER, 2004).

Grapes are considered to be one of the greatest sources of phenolic compounds when compared to other fruits and vegetables. Grape seeds and skins contain flavonoids (catechin, epicatechin, procyanidins and anthocyanins), phenolic acids and resveratrol, which have been shown to have functional activities. The procyanidin extract from grape seeds showed antioxidant activity. As grapes are part of our diet and are rich in phenolic compounds, studying their antioxidant activity is extremely important (SATO et al., 2001).

Watermelon (*Citrullus lanatus*), which originated in the dry regions of tropical Africa, is the most widely produced *cucurbitaceous plant* in the world. Watermelon is a source of minerals (potassium, magnesium, calcium and iron) and amino acids (citrulline and arginine), as well as being rich in compounds with antioxidant properties such as lycopene, vitamin C, flavonoids and other phenolic compounds (WHO-OLIU et al., 2012; RAWSON et al., 2011). Its consumption has been associated with the prevention of degenerative diseases such as prostate, stomach and lung cancer, the treatment of diabetes mellitus, metabolic syndrome and the reduction of blood pressure (AHN et al., 2011; WU et al., 2007; FIGUEROA et al.,

2012).

According to Dias et al. (2006), watermelon has pleasant sensory characteristics of aroma, color, flavor and refreshment. The pulp and rind are used to produce flours, dehydrated products, jams, jellies, cakes, cookies and juices on an artisanal or low-industrial scale. Watermelon is one of the fruits with a high water content and which produces a large amount of waste such as peel, skin and seeds. It is important to emphasize the need for watermelon processing as a way of making use of waste and reducing waste due to its high perfectibility (SILVA et al., 2010; RAWSON et al., 2011; GUIMARAES; FREITAS; SILVA, 2010).

Passion fruit (*Passiflora edulis Sims*) belongs to the *Passifloraceae* family, whose main species of economic importance is *Passiflora edulis Sims*, known as yellow passion fruit. Passion fruit can be used for fresh consumption, however, its greatest economic importance lies in its use for industrial purposes, processing to make whole juice, nectar and concentrated juice. Juice is widely consumed because of its nutritional value and excellent organoleptic characteristics, making it the second largest seller on the domestic market. The peel and dry extract of passion fruit have been used to lower glucose levels in diabetes, exerting a positive effect on glycemic control. The probable mechanism for this action is present in the fruit's peel, which has a high content of pectin, a water-soluble dietary fiber that helps lower blood glucose and cholesterol levels. Adding dietary fiber to the diet improves glucose tolerance in diabetic patients treated with insulin or not (RAVAZZI, 2004). Contraindications: Its use is contraindicated during pregnancy. Do not use in cases of treatment with sedatives or nervous system depressants (BRASIL, 2011).

Many functional properties of passion fruit peel have been studied in recent years, especially those related to the content and type of fibers present. Passion fruit peel, which accounts for 52% of the fruit's chemical composition, can no longer be considered industrial waste, since its characteristics and functional properties can be used to develop new products (MEDINA, 1980). Oral dosage for adolescents and adults: infuse 1-2 g of the plant drug in 150 mL of boiling water, take 1-4 times a day (10-15 minutes after preparation), while the encapsulated plant drug: 0.5-2 g, 1-4 times a day (EMA, 2014). Fluid extract: (1:1 in 25% ethyl alcohol) - 0.5 to 1.0 mL, 3 times a day. Tincture: (1:8 in 45% alcohol) - 0.5 to 2.0 mL, 3 times a day (MÜLLER et al., 2005). The recommended dosage for adults is 3-5 times a day, and for adolescents 3 times a day (EMA, 2014). The dose of the dry extract should correspond to the dosage of the forms described above.

Other functional foods can be cited from plant sources that reduce the risk of chronic diseases, particularly cancer, and provide health benefits for the individual. These include: garlic, tomatoes, onions, cabbage, cauliflower, broccoli, green or black tea, soybeans, oats, citrus fruits and flax seeds (SGARBIERI, 2002).

4 CONCLUSIONS

In this context, we can conclude that phytotherapy is an area of extreme importance both as a natural therapy and as a nutritional therapy. As a natural therapy, it stands out for being a simple and natural treatment, more accessible, low-cost and with low side effects, as it is an effective form of primary health care, complementing the drug treatment usually used by the poor. Nutritional therapy through phytotherapy has been gaining ground in relation to foods and their functional properties, preventing diseases and providing a better quality of life for the population. According to CFN Resolution No. 556 of April 11, 2015, the practice of phytotherapy by professional nutritionists to complement dietary prescriptions is regulated.

REFERENCES

AHN, J. et al. Anti-diabetic effect of watermelon (*Citrullus vulgaris* Schrad) on streptozotocin-induceddiabetic mice. **Food Science and Biotechnology**, v. 20, n. 1, p. 251-254, 2011.

ALONSO, J. R. **Tratado de fitomedicina: bases clinicas y farmacológicas**. Buenos Aires: Editora Isis, 1998.

ALVIN, N. A. T. et al. The use of medicinal plants as a therapeutic resource: from the influences of professional training to the ethical and legal implications of its applicability as an extension of the nurse's care practice.

Revista Latino Americana de Enfermagem, v. 14, n. 3, p. 316-323, 2006.

ARAÙJO, A. A. **Medicina rùstica**. 3ª ed. Sao Paulo: Brasiliense, 2007.

ARRUDA, J. T. et al. Effect of aqueous extract of chamomile (*Chamomilla recutita* L.) on rat pregnancy and pup development. **Revista Brasileira de Plantas Medicinais**, v. 15, p. 66-71, 2013.

BRAGANÇA, L. A. R. **Antidiabetic medicinal plants: A multidisciplinary approach.** Rio de Janeiro: Editora EDUFF, 1996.

BRAZIL. National Health Surveillance Agency. **Formulary of Herbal Medicines from the Brazilian Pharmacopoeia**. F ed. Brasilia, DF: Anvisa, 2011. 126 p.

CECHINEL-FILHO, V.; YUNES, R.A. Strategies for obtaining pharmacologically active compounds from medicinal plants: concepts on structural modification to optimize activity. **Quimica Nova**, v. 21, n. 1, p. 99-105, 1998.

CORDEIRO, R.; NUNES, V.; ALMEIDA, C. R. **Enciclopédia das plantas que curam: a natureza a serviço de sua saù**. Sao Paulo: Grupo de Comunicaçao

Três S/A, 1996.

DIAS, R. C. S. et al. Agronomic performance of watermelon lines with resistance to oidium. **Horticultura Brasileira**, v. 24, p.1416-1418, 2006.

DINIZ, R. C. Municipal Phytotherapy Program in the municipality of Londrina, Paranâ. **Saùde Debate**, n.34, p.73-80, 2006.

D'IPPOLITO, J. A. C.; ROCHA, L. M.; SILVA, R. F. **Fitoterapia Magistral: A practical guide to the handling of herbal** medicines. Sâo Paulo: Anfarmag, 194p, 2005.

EMA. European Medicines Agency**. Community herbal monograph on *Passiflora incarnata***, herba, 2014.

FERREIRA, T. S. et al. Phytotherapy: an introduction to its history, use and application. **Revista Brasileira de Plantas Medicinais**, v.16, n. 2, p. 290-298, 2014.

FIGUEROA, A. et al. Watermelon extract supplementation reduces ankle blood pressure and carotid augmentation index in obese adults with prehypertension or hypertension. **American Journal of Hypertension**, v. 25, n. 6, p. 640-643, 2012.

GUIMARAES, R. R.; FREITAS, M. C. J.; SILVA, V.L.M. Simple cakes made with watermelon peel flour (*Citrullus vulgaris*, sobral): chemical, physical and sensory evaluation. **Ciência e Tecnologia de Alimentos**, v. 30, n. 2, p. 354-363, 2010.

LIMA, A.; LOPPES, A. H. N. **indice Terapèutico Fitoterâpico**. 1ª ed. Petrópolis, RJ: EPUB, 328p, 2008.

MARTINAZZO, A. P.; MARTINS, T. Plantas medicinais utilizados pela populaçâo de Cascavel/PR. **Arquivo de Ciências e Saùde da Unipar**, v. 8, n. 1, p. 3-5, 2004.

MATOS, F. J. A. **Farmâcias vivas - A system for using medicinal plants designed for small communities**. 4th ed. Fortaleza: EUFC, 267p, 2002.

MEDINA, J.C. **Some technological aspects of tropical fruits and their products.** Sâo Paulo: Secretaria de Agricultura e Abastecimento de Sâo Paulo. 295p, 1980.

MÜLLER, S. D. et al. LC and UV determination of flavonoids from Passiflora alata medicinal extracts and leaves. **Journal of Pharmaceutical and Biomedical Analysis**, v. 37, p. 399-403, 2005.

OLIVEIRA, M. J. R; SIMOES, M. J. S; SASSI, C.R.R. Phytotherapy in the public health system (SUS) in the State of Sao Paulo, Brazil. **Revista Brasileira de Plantas Medicinais**, v. 8, n. 2, p. 39-41, 2006.

OMS-OLIU, G. et al. Stability of health-related compounds in plant foods through the application of non-thermal. **Trends in Food Science and Technology**, v. 23, p. 111-123, 2012.

PINTO, E. P. P.; AMOROZO, M. C. M.; FURLAN, A. Popular knowledge of medicinal plants in rural communities in the Atlantic Forest - Itacaré, BA, Brazil. **Acta Botànica Brasilica**, v. 20, n. 4, p. 751-762, 2006.

RAVAZZI, E. F. R. **The use of passiflora sp. in the control of diabetes mellitus: a preliminary qualitative study**. 2004. Monograph (Degree in Pharmacy).

University Center of Maringà, 2004.

RAWSON, A. et al. Effect of thermosonication on bioactive compounds in water melon juice. **Food Research International**, v. 44, p. 1168-1173, 2011.

ROSA, R. L.; BARCELOS, A. L. V.; BAMPI, G. Investigation of the use of medicinal plants in the treatment of individuals with diabetes mellitus in the city of Herval D' Oeste - SC. **Revista Brasileira de Plantas Medicinais**, v. 14, n. 2, p. 306-310, 2012.

SATO, M. et al. Grape seed proanthocyanidin reduces cardiomyocyte apoptosis by inhibiting ischemia/reperfusion-induced activation of JNK-1 and C-JUN. **Free Radical Biology and Medicine**, v. 31, n. 6, p. 729-737, 2001.

SCHULZ, V.; HANSEL, R.; TYLER, V. E. **Rational Phytotherapy**, 4ª ed., Sao Paulo: Editora Manole, 2002.

SCHLEIER, R. **Phytochemical constituents of *Vitis viniferal* (grape)**. Monograph presented to obtain the title of Specialist in Phytotherapy at IBEHE/FACIS. Sao Paulo: IBEHE, 2004.

SGARBIERI, V. Awareness that diseases begin in the womb increases demand for functional foods. **Jornal da Unicamp**, Sao Paulo, November 2002.

SILVA, E. L. et al. Acute ingestion of yerba mate infusion (Ilex paraguariensis) inhibits plasma and lipoprotein oxidation. **Food Research International**, v. 41, p. 973-979, 2010.

SIMOES, C. M. O.; SCHENKEL, E. P. **Plantas da Medicina Popular do Rio Grande do Sul**. 5th ed., Porto Alegre: Editora da UFRGS, 2011.

SINGI, G. et al. Acute effects of hydroalcoholic extracts of garlic (*Allium sativum* L.) and lemongrass (*Cymbopogon citratus* (DC) Stapf) on mean arterial pressure of anesthetized rats. **Revista Brasileira de Farmacognosia**, v. 15, n. 2, p. 94-97, 2005.

TOMAZZONI, M. I.; NEGRELLE, R. R. B.; CENTA, M. Popular phytotherapy: the instrumental search as a therapeutic practice. **Texto Contexto Enfermagem**, v. 15, n. 1, p. 115-21, 2006.

VANACLOCHA, B.V.; FOLCARA, S. C. **Fitoterapia: Vademécum de Prescripción**, 4ª ed., Barcelona: Masson, 1091p, 2003.

WHO. WORLD HEALTH ORGANIZATION. **WHO monographs on selected medicinal plants.** Geneva, Switzerland: World Health Organization, v. 1, p. 86-94, 1999.

WU, G. et al. Dietary supplementation with watermelon pomace juice enhances arginine availability and ameliorates the metabolic syndrome in zucker diabetic fatty rats. **The Journal of Nutrition**, v. 137, p. 2680-2685, 2007.

CHAPTER 5

THE IMPORTANCE OF MEDICINAL PLANTS IN DIABETES MELLITUS TYPE II: A REVIEW

Ana Priscila Silva Moreno[1]

Wlliane Silva Soares[1]

Maria das Graças Silva[2]

1. Postgraduate student in Clinical and Functional Nutrition at Faculdade Integrada de Patos;

2. Master's Degree in Natural and Synthetic Bioactive Products, Federal University of Paraiba.

SUMMARY: Diabetes mellitus is a group of diseases characterized by high blood glucose concentrations resulting from defects in insulin secretion, insulin action or both. Diabetes is a serious problem worldwide and affects thousands of people. In developing countries, there is a tendency for its frequency to increase in all age groups, especially the younger ones, whose negative impact on quality of life and the burden of the disease on health systems is immeasurable. Population ageing and changes in lifestyle are identified as the main determinants of the sharp increase in the frequency of type 2 diabetes mellitus in recent years. Medicinal plants have therefore emerged as a topic of great interest in the treatment of diabetes, due to their hypoglycemic properties. Therefore, the aim of this study was to present the potential of popularly used plants in the treatment of diabetes, to focus on nutritional and pharmacological therapy, to verify the main therapeutic effects of medicinal plants and to identify the chemical substances of plants with therapeutic action in type II diabetes mellitus. The study was characterized by exploratory bibliographical research. It was concluded that most of the plants used as antidiabetics, when evaluated pharmacologically, demonstrate hypoglycemic activity and have chemical constituents that can be used as models for new hypoglycemic agents, such as *Bauhinia fortificata*, *Allium sativum* L., *Allium cepa* L. and *Anacardium occidentale*. The search for plants or natural compounds with antidiabetic activity meets the need for new active compounds that are less toxic and possibly more accessible to the population.

Keywords: Diabetes mellitus. Medicinal plants. Treatment.

1 INTRODUCTION

Diabetes mellitus is a group of diseases characterized by elevated blood glucose concentrations resulting from defects in insulin secretion, insulin action or both (FRANZ, 2012).

In many countries, the prevalence of type 2 diabetes mellitus has risen dramatically, and is expected to rise even further. In developing countries, there is a tendency for the frequency to increase in all age groups, especially the younger ones, whose negative impact on quality of life and the burden of the disease on health systems is immeasurable (SARTORELLI; FRANCO; CARDOSO, 2006).

Population aging and lifestyle changes have been identified as the main determinants of the sharp increase in the frequency of type 2 diabetes mellitus in recent years, which can be substantiated by the alarming prevalence of altered glucose homeostasis (GH) among genetically susceptible individuals exposed to drastic changes in eating behavior and physical activity.

Currently, type 2 diabetes mellitus (DM2) is considered to be one of the main chronic diseases affecting contemporary man, affecting populations in countries at all stages of biological and economic-social development. Among children and adolescents, some factors have been consistently recognized as being associated with DM2. These include: family history of DM2, obesity, sedentary lifestyle, hypertension, age, gender and high capillary blood glucose levels.

Most of the plants used as antidiabetic agents, when evaluated pharmacologically, have been shown to have hypoglycemic activity and chemical constituents that can be used as models for new hypoglycemic agents, such as: Cow's foot (*Bauhinia fortificata)*, Garlic (*Allium sativum* L.), Onion (*Allium cepa* L.) and Cashew (*Anacardium occidentale*).

Therefore, the general objective of this study was to carry out a bibliographical survey of medicinal plants used in the treatment of type 2 diabetes mellitus. specific objectives were to focus on nutritional and pharmacological therapy, to verify the main therapeutic effects of medicinal plants and to identify the chemical substances of plants with therapeutic action in type 2 diabetes mellitus.

2 MATERIAL AND METHODS

The study was characterized by exploratory research in terms of objectives and bibliographic research in terms of data collection procedures. The survey was carried out by searching electronic databases such as Medline, Scielo and Periódicos CAPES.

Exploratory research is often the first stage of a broader investigation; among exploratory research is bibliographical research, which is carried out using material that has already been prepared, consisting mainly of books and scientific articles (SANTOS, 2004; GIL, 2011).

In order to achieve the objectives, the bibliographical research was carried out in the following stages: choice of topic, preliminary survey, formulation of the problem, elaboration of the problem, elaboration of the provisional plan of the subject, search for sources, reading of the material, logical organization of the subject and writing of the text for the conclusion of the research.

3 Results and discussion

3.1 Concepts of Diabetes Mellitus

Diabetes Mellitus is a chronic, hereditary disease characterized by an abnormal rise in blood glucose levels, known as hyperglycemia, and by the excretion of excess glucose in the urine, known as glycosuria. The basic defect seems to be an absolute or relative lack of insulin, or a decrease in the insulin receptors on the membrane of the target cells, which leads to alterations in the metabolism of glucose, proteins and fats (ANDERSON et al., 1998).

Diabetes mellitus is a metabolic disease characterized by excess glucose in the blood and eventually in the urine (GROSSI, 2009). It is an endocrine disorder that consists of a defect in the secretion and/or action of insulin produced by the pancreas, manifested by the inadequate use of glucose by the tissues, which causes hyperglycemia (SBD, 2013).

According to Ferreira (2003), it is a chronic, heterogeneous disease characterized by alterations in carbohydrate metabolism, which result in absolute insulin deficiency. Generally, protein and lipid metabolism are affected, leading to ketosis and acidosis, and the diagnostic marker is persistent chronic hyperglycemia.

With the decline in infectious and parasitic diseases, there have been epidemiological changes such as an increase in the incidence of morbidity and mortality from chronic non-communicable diseases (CNCDs), including diabetes (GRILLO; GORINI, 2007).

The pancreas is made up of two organs, the endocrine and the exocrine. The endocrine organ is responsible for producing the hormone insulin, among others, and any alteration in this organ results in damage to the body (OKOSHI et al., 2007).

Glucose is the main signal for the pancreas to release insulin through the β cells of the islets of Langerhans (GUYTON; HALL, 2012). The cells have insulin receptors, insulin binds to the receptors and mobilizes the glucose transporters (GLUT), in the adipose tissue there is GLUT 4, in the pancreas there is GLUT 2. The GLUTs go to the surface of the cells and transport glucose into the cells (COTRAN; KUMAR; COLLINS, 2010).

Most of the glucose goes into the glycolytic pathway, where it is transformed into glycogen (glucose stock). In situations of prolonged fasting and diabetes, the cells are short of glucose and triglycerides are broken down to obtain energy (AZEVEDO; GROSS, 1990 apud ALMINO; QUEIROZ; JORGE, 2009).

3.2 Classification

Diabetes mellitus can be classified into two forms: insulin-dependent diabetes mellitus and non-insulin-dependent diabetes mellitus, i.e. type 1 and type 2 diabetes. Type 1 diabetes accounts for 5% of all known cases, usually children, adolescents or adults up to the age of 30 who are thin, prone to ketoacidosis and dependent on exogenous insulin. Type 2 diabetes, on the other hand, accounts for 90% of diabetes cases and generally affects adults aged over 30, who are obese (around 80% are android-type obese) and do not depend on insulin for glycemic control (FERREIRA, 2003).

The two most common types are type 1 and type 2 and both have impaired regulation of blood glucose by insulin. Diabetic individuals have an increased risk of suffering a cardiovascular event and double the risk of dying from this event when compared to the general population (SBD, 2013).

3.2.1 Type 1 diabetes mellitus

At the time of diagnosis, individuals with type 1 diabetes mellitus are usually thin and may present with excessive thirst, frequent urination and significant weight loss. The primary defect is the destruction of pancreatic β-cells, leading to absolute insulin deficiency and, consequently, hyperglycemia, polyuria (excessive urination), polydipsia (excessive thirst), weight loss, dehydration, electrolyte disturbance and ketoacidosis (FRANZ, 2012).

In type 1 diabetes mellitus, the disease is usually caused by an autoimmune process and results from the destruction of the beta cells of the pancreas, leading to an absolute insulin deficiency (GREENSPAN; STREWLER, 2006).

In symptomatic patients, polyuria, polyphagia, polydipsia, weight loss and visual changes are common. In addition, patients can suffer chronic complications such as atherosclerosis, myocardial infarction and become more susceptible to infections such as carbuncles and generalized furunculosis. In these patients, insulin administration is necessary to avoid the development of ketoacidosis, coma and death (FIGUEIREDO; RABELO, 2009).

Type 1 diabetes is common in children and young adults, and insulin replacement is the only form of treatment for these cases (GOMEZ; VENTURINI, 2009).

3.2.2 Type 2 diabetes mellitus

Type 2 diabetes mellitus accounts for 90% to 95% of all diagnosed cases of diabetes and is a progressive disease which, in many cases, is present long before it is diagnosed. Hyperglycemia develops gradually and is almost always not severe enough in the early stages for the patient to notice any of the classic symptoms of diabetes. Although undiagnosed, these individuals are likely to develop macro- and microvascular complications (FRANZ, 2012).

Type 2 comprises a more heterogeneous group of milder forms of the disease, which occurs predominantly in adults and can begin in childhood. It accounts for approximately 90% of diabetes cases worldwide and is characterized by insulin resistance and/or reduced insulin secretion (GREENSPAN; STREWLER, 2006).

Type 2 diabetes is caused by insulin resistance and obesity and affects people over the age of 40. The pancreas secretes insulin normally, but there is too much insulin and too little glucose in the blood. The pancreas releases too much insulin, causing the β-cells to deteriorate. Destroyed β-cells produce no insulin and the individual needs to take insulin and medication to increase insulin sensitivity (GUYTON; HALL, 2012).

It is characterized by insulin resistance and can progress to insulin deficiency. It usually occurs in obese patients over the age of 35 and can be associated with hypertension and atherosclerosis. For these type 2 patients, treatment with oral hypoglycemic agents aims to reduce insulin resistance and stimulate insulin secretion (GOMEZ; VENTURINI, 2009).

In type 2 diabetes (non-insulin-dependent diabetes), the pancreas continues to produce insulin, sometimes at higher levels than normal. However, the body develops a resistance to its effects and the result is a relative insulin deficit (COTRAN; KUMAR; COLLINS, 2010).

3.3 Nutritional Therapy in Diabetes Mellitus

According to Sachs (2002), the main objective of nutritional self-control is to help people with diabetes keep their blood glucose as close to normal as possible, balancing diet, medication and physical exercise. It's important to note that not all diet plans are necessarily restricted in terms of energy. Children, adolescents, pregnant women and nursing mothers need enough energy to ensure that they perform well in each specific state. Malnourished people should also receive adequate energy to recover their nutritional status.

According to Franz (2012), nutritional therapy is a fundamental part of diabetes treatment and care. Integrating NT into overall diabetes treatment effectively requires a coordinated team effort, which must include a nutritionist, who has the knowledge and skills to implement current principles and recommendations for diabetes.

Diet therapy in diabetes mellitus aims to reduce blood glucose to normal levels or as close to them as possible, to reduce the effects of the disease, maintaining a normal metabolic state (normal blood glucose, lipids and amino acids), to prevent acute and chronic complications, to promote lifestyle changes (smoking cessation, increased physical activity, and reorganization of eating habits) according to needs, always respecting dietary preferences and socioeconomic status. In this way, the risk of acute decompensation due to diabetic ketoacidosis or hyperglycemic non-ketotic hyperosmolar syndrome is greatly reduced; the symptoms of blurred vision are relieved, the risk of polyuria, fatigue, polydipsia, weight loss with polyphagia is reduced and the risks of the onset and/or progression of nephropathy, morbidity and mortality and diabetic retinopathy, which is known as a prolonged excess of sugar in the blood, are reduced; the blood vessels of the retina become more permeable, allowing the leakage of blood and fluid: called edema. As a result, diabetic retinopathy sufferers may initially notice blurred vision and the condition may progress to partial or even total loss of vision (FERREIRA, 2003).

Depending on the patient's needs, the goals of therapy can be achieved by diet; diet plus insulin; or diet plus oral hypoglycemic agents. In obese diabetics without symptoms, both hyperglycemia and hyperinsulinemia can be corrected by a calorie-restricted diet, which results in weight loss or growth, combined with daily insulin injections. Obese diabetics with symptoms usually respond to a calorie-restricted diet to promote weight loss and an oral hypoglycemic agent. However, some patients in the latter group may require insulin to treat the disease (ANDERSON et al., 1998).

A diabetic's diet should be individualized according to daily calorie needs, physical activity and eating habits. In non-diabetics, calorie expenditure is calculated as 30 to 40 calories/kg/day. In obese T2DM, which occurs in 85 to 90% of cases, the daily calorie intake should be reduced by 15 to 30% or more. This alone would reduce three of the risk factors for cardiovascular disease: obesity, dyslipidemia (present in around a third of diabetics) and hypertension. A low-calorie diet alone improves insulin sensitivity and reduces hyperglycemia, regardless of weight loss (ARAÙJO; BRITTO; CRUZ, 2000).

According to Gomez and Venturini (2009), basic dietary care for diabetics includes the consumption of foods rich in fiber such as whole grains, peeled fruits and vegetables, as these slow down the intestinal absorption of glucose, promoting the maintenance of intestinal flora and, consequently, the synthesis of vitamin B12 in the colon. In addition, some foods with antioxidant properties are recommended, such as those rich in copper, zinc, chromium, magnesium, vitamins E, C and A. This is because it is known that chronic hyperglycemia promotes an imbalance, known as oxidative stress, which is responsible for vascular microlesions and the appearance of glaucoma, diabetic foot, hypertension, kidney failure and other complications associated with diabetes. Therefore, the consumption of foods with antioxidant properties can minimize or delay the appearance of such damage.

Nutritional therapy is the first treatment option for most pregnant women with gestational diabetes. This therapy avoids excessive weight gain in pregnant women, as well as generating a lower rate of fetal macrosomia and perinatal complications (SARTORI et al., 2006).

Carbohydrate intake should be restricted to less than 42% of daily calories, with the rest distributed between proteins and fats, as evidence shows that pregnant women who restrict their intake in this way have better postprandial glycemic control, less need for insulin, a lower incidence of fetal macrosomia and caesarean section (RUDGE et al., 2005). In addition, complex carbohydrates with a low glycemic index (pasta, wholemeal bread and cereals with a high fiber content) should be prioritized.

The total caloric value of the diet is distributed over three meals and two to three snacks. In obese pregnant women, snacks can be eliminated (BRASIL, 2010).

Breakfast should contain around 10% of the day's calories; lunch, 30%; dinner, 30%; and snacks, 30%. Very restrictive diets (less than 1,500 kcal/day) can induce ketonemia and are not recommended (RUDGE et al., 2005).

Diets with moderate calorie restriction (1,600 - 1,800 kcal) do not lead to ketosis and are effective in controlling maternal weight gain and glycemic control. Reducing calories in the diet by 50% has similar benefits to reducing it by 33% for glycemic control; the latter does not lead to ketosis and is therefore the recommended restriction (RUDGE et al., 2005). The minimum carbohydrate intake recommended during pregnancy is 175 g per day (COTRAN; KUMAR; COLLINS, 2010).

Nutritional treatment of patients with diabetes aims to achieve the following goals: a) provide all essential elements (e.g. vitamins and minerals); b) achieve and maintain a reasonable weight; c) meet energy needs; d) avoid large daily fluctuations in blood glucose levels, with levels as close to normal as possible, as well as practice and decrease blood lipid levels, if elevated (COTRAN; KUMAR; COLLINS, 2010).

It is worth noting that for all diabetic patients, the meal plan should take into account their food preferences, lifestyle, usual meal times and ethnic and cultural background (SARTORI et al., 2006). For patients using intensive insulin therapy regimens, there can be greater flexibility in the timing and content of meals by making adjustments for changes in eating and exercise habits (COSTA et al., 2003).

3.4 Pharmacological therapy

3.4.1 Insulin

Insulin is a hormone produced by specialized cells located in the islets of Langherans in the pancreas (GOMEZ; VENTURINI, 2009).

The indication for insulin in the treatment of DM2 is reserved for symptomatic diabetics with severe hyperglycemia, ketonemia or ketonuria, even if they are newly diagnosed, or for diabetics who do not respond to treatment with diet, exercise and/or oral hypoglycemic agents, antihyperglycemic agents or insulin action sensitizers (ARAÙJO; BRITTO; CRUZ, 2000).

According to Gomez and Venturini (2009), insulin for clinical use has been extracted from the pancreas of cattle and pigs and, more recently, human insulin has been cloned using biotechnological techniques. Pharmacological manipulations allow insulin to be presented in its natural, soluble form or as small crystals of different sizes, producing fast-acting, intermediate or slow-acting forms. The route of insulin administration can be intramuscular, intravenous or, more commonly, subcutaneous. It cannot be administered orally, as the gastric pH completely destroys this hormone.

3.4.2 Hypoglycemic Agents and Food Interactions

Drug interactions are special types of pharmacological responses, in which the effects of one or more drugs are altered by the simultaneous or previous administration of others, or through concurrent administration with food (SECOLI, 2001).

In addition to all the nutritional care required for glycemic and weight control in diabetic patients, some drugs have important interactions with nutrients. Metformin, a member of the biguanide class, causes vitamin B12 (cyanocobalamin) deficiency in around 30% of patients. Although few cases of megaloblastic anemia have been attributed to vitamin B12 deficiency due to treatment with metformin, caution should be exercised as signs of deficiency can be confused with peripheral neuropathy, which is common in diabetic patients. If levels of this vitamin are low, it may be useful to increase the frequency of consumption of foods such as liver steak, millet, shellfish and oysters, which are the main sources of vitamin B12, as well as foods of animal origin in general (GOMEZ; VENTURINI, 2009).

3.5 Phytotherapy

The aim of herbal medicine is not to replace medicines registered and marketed by laboratories, but rather to act as an optional form of therapy, under the care of professionals who care for the illness, considering that it is a lower cost treatment and the benefits will be added to conventional therapy (SILVA et al., 2008).

The demand for less expensive therapies for the treatment of chronic degenerative diseases represents an important gain in human and financial investment in the health sector. The use of herbal medicines is intended to act as an optional form of therapy available to professionals who care for diabetic patients (CAVALLI et al., 2007).

Phytotherapy uses the various parts of plants, such as roots, bark, leaves, fruit and seeds, depending on the herb in question. There are also different ways of preparing these plants, the most commonly used being tea, prepared by decoction or infusion. In the first process, the plant to be used is boiled together with water, while in the second, the water is boiled alone and then placed on the plant, when its therapeutic principles are released (REZENDE; COCCO, 2002).

3.6 Medicinal plants

Plants are natural laboratories where a large number of chemical products are biosynthesized, and are considered to be the most important source of chemical compounds in existence. A large percentage of the active ingredients are in the so-called natural products or secondary metabolites, which are chemical compounds with relatively complex structures and restricted distribution. These metabolites have common defensive functions against insects, bacteria and fungi, such as alkaloids, non-protein amino acids, steroids, phenols, flavonoids, coumarins, quinones, tannins and terpenoids. There is considerable variation in their concentration in the plant, i.e. higher concentrations of these types of compounds are found in leaves, flowers and seeds (AGUILAR et al., 2012).

Medicinal plants have multiple benefits, such as the control of carbohydrate metabolism, through various mechanisms such as the prevention and

restoring the integrity and function of pancreatic β-cells, stimulating the release of insulin, improving the uptake and utilization of glucose and their antioxidant properties, making plants an excellent target for the development of new therapeutic models (ROCHA et al., 2006).

Also according to Rocha et al. (2006), natural antioxidant substances with hypoglycemic activity are potential therapeutic agents in the prevention and treatment of diabetes complications.

Most of the plants used as antidiabetics have been pharmacologically evaluated and shown to have hypoglycemic activity and chemical constituents that can be used as models for new hypoglycemic agents (SILVA et al., 2008).

3.7 Medicinal plants used in type II diabetes mellitus

3.7.1 Cow paw (*Bauhinia fortificata*)

It is an evergreen tree that adapts to any soil planting, requiring full light. It is planted from seed. The leaves in particular are considered antidiabetic and are used in home medicine to treat other illnesses (SILVA et al., 2008).

Cow's foot (*Bauhinia forficata*) has long been used in folk medicine to treat diabetes. The decoction can be used to treat diabetes because it improves the condition without causing detectable tissue toxicity (SPETHMANN, 2004).

According to Silva and Cechinel Filho (2002), in Brazil plants of the genus Bauhinia are known as "Pata-de-vaca" or "Unha-de-boi". The leaves, stems and roots of *Bauhinia* species, especially *B. manca*, *B. rufescens*, *B. forficata*, *B. cheitantha*, and *B. splendens*, are widely used in Brazil and other countries in the form of teas and other herbal preparations for the treatment of various ailments, especially infections, painful processes and diabetes.

Its chemical constituents are tannins, steroids, pinitol, choline, trigonelline, glycosides, rhamnosides, astragoline, flavanoids, and mucilage, in which the whole plant is used (CORRÊA; BATISTA; QUINTAS, 2011).

3.7.2 Garlic (*Allium sativum* L.) and Onion (*Allium cepa* L.)

Popularly known as garlic, it is a plant widely used both in traditional medicine and as a condiment. It is popularly used to treat cardiovascular diseases, as an antithrombotic, antidiabetic, antimicrobial, antitumor and lipid-lowering agent (SEMGUPTA; GHOSH; BHATTACHARJEE, 2004).

Different studies indicate that garlic (*Allium sativum* L.) helps stabilize blood sugar levels (SPETHMANN, 2004).

According to Zaparolli et al. (2013), onions (*Allium cepa* L.) and garlic (*Allium sativum* L.) are foods widely used for medicinal applications. They are sources of numerous phytochemicals used in the treatment and prevention of various diseases, including cancer, coronary heart disease, obesity, hypercholesterolemia, diabetes, hypertension and disorders of the gastrointestinal tract. Garlic has a considerable content of selenium, which acts as an antioxidant, and alliin, which has a hypotensive and hypoglycemic action. Onions are rich in the flavonoid quercetin, which has health-related properties due to its high antioxidant power.

According to Corrêa, Batista and Quintas (2011), garlic's chemical composition includes allicin, deoxyalliin, vinyl polysulphides, allyl, diallyl and allylpropyl, while onions contain vitamins A, B1, B2, B5, C, mineral salts (potassium, phosphorus, calcium, sodium, silicon, magnesium, iron) and glycoquinine, and the bulbs are mainly used.

3.7.3 Cashew tree (*Anacardium occidentale*)

Popularly known through its fruit, which is widely consumed throughout the country, the nut is very popular and exported to almost the entire world. Its chemical composition contains carotenes, vitamin C, phenolic acids, terpenes, flavonoids, tannins, aromatic substances (anacardic acid, anacardol, cardol) and resins (acajucica). The bark, leaves, flowers and fruit are used (SILVA et al., 2008).

4 CONCLUSIONS

Diabetes mellitus is a serious public health problem due to its high prevalence in the population, its chronic complications, mortality, the high financial and social costs involved in treatment and the significant deterioration in quality of life. Most of the plants used as antidiabetics have been pharmacologically evaluated and shown to have hypoglycemic activity and chemical constituents that can be used as models for new hypoglycemic agents, such as *Bauhinia fortificata*, *Allium sativum* L., *Allium cepa* L., *Anacardium occidentale*.

The aim of herbal medicine is not to replace medicines registered and marketed by laboratories, but rather to act as an optional form of therapy, under the care of professionals who treat the illness, considering that it is a lower-cost treatment and the benefits will be added to conventional therapy.

The search for plants or natural compounds with antidiabetic activity meets the need for new active compounds that are less toxic and possibly more accessible to the population.

REFERENCES

AGUILAR, Y. M et al. Secondary metabolites and in vitro antidiabetic activity of *Anacardium occidentale* L. (cashew) leaf extracts. **Revista Cubana Medicina da Planta**, v. 17, n. 4, p. 320-329, 2012.

ALMINO, M. A. F. B.; QUEIROZ, M. V. O.; JORGE, M. S. B. Diabetes mellitus in adolescence: experiences and feelings of adolescents and mothers with the disease. **Revista de Enfermagem da USP**, v. 43, n. 4, p. 760-767, 2009.

ANDERSON, L. et al. Diabetes Mellitus. In: **Nutrition**. Rio de Janeiro: Guanabara, ch. 19, p.443, 1998.

ARAÙJO, L. M. B.; BRITTO, M. M. S.; CRUZ, T. R. P. Treatment of Type 2 Diabetes Mellitus: New Options. **Arquivos Brasileiros de Endocrinologia e Metabologia**, v.44, n. 6, p. 509-518, 2000.

BRAZIL. Ministry of Health. Health Care Secretariat. Department of Strategic Programmatic Actions. **High-risk pregnancy: Technical Manual.** Ministry of Health, Secretariat of Health Care, Department of Strategic Programmatic Actions. 5ª ed. Brasilia: Editora do Ministério da Saùde, 2010. p 302.

CAVALLI, V. L. et al. In vivo evaluation of the hypoglycemic effect of extracts obtained from the root and leaf of burdock *Arctium minus* (Hill.) Bernh. **Brazilian Journal of Pharmacognosy**, v. 17, n. 1, p. 64-70, 2007.

CORRÊA, A. D.; BATISTA, R. S.; QUINTAS, L. E. M. **Plantas Medicinais do cultivo à terapêutica**. 8th ed. Rio de Janeiro: Petrópolis, p. 75-108, 2011.

COSTA, A. C. F. et al. Analysis of diagnostic criteria for glucose metabolism disorders and variables associated with insulin resistance. **Brazilian Journal of Pathology and Laboratory Medicine**, v. 39, n. 2. p. 125-130, 2003.

COTRAN, R. S.; KUMAR, V.; COLLINS, T. **Robbins: structural and functional pathology.** 8th ed. Rio de Janeiro: Guanabara Koogan, 2010.

FERREIRA, T. R. A. S. Diabetes Mellitus. In: TEXEIRA, N. F. **Nutriçâo Clinica.** Rio de Janeiro: Guanabara Koogan, chap. 38, p. 408-411, 2003.

FIGUEIREDO, D. M.; RABELO, F. L. A. Diabetes *insipidus*: main aspects and comparative analysis with diabetes mellitus. **Seminàrio Ciências Biológicas da Saùde**, v. 30, n. 2, p. 155-162, 2009.

FRANZ, M. J. Clinical Nutritional Therapy for Diabetes Mellitus and Hypoglycemia of Non-Diabetic Origin. In: MAHAN, L. K.; ESCOTT-STUMP, S.; RAYMOND, J. L. **Krause: Food, Nutrition and Diet Therapy.** Rio de Janeiro: Elsevier, ch. 31, p. 675-683, 2012.

GIL, A. C. **Métodos e Técnicas de Pesquisa Social.** 6th ed. Sâo Paulo, Editora: Atlas, chap. 6, p. 49-59, 2011.

GOMEZ, R.; VENTURINI, C. D. **Interaçâo entre alimentos e medicamentos.** Porto Alegre: Letra e Vida, 168p, 2009.

GREENSPAN, F.; STREWLER, G. **Basic & Clinical Endocrinology**. 7ª ed. Rio de Janeiro: Guanabara Koogan, 599p, 2006.

GRILLO, M. F. F.; GORINI, M. I. P. C. Characterization of people with Type 2 Diabetes Mellitus. **Revista Brasileira de Enfermagem**, v. 60, n. 1, p. 49-54, 2007.

GROSSI, S. A. A. Managing Diabetes Mellitus from the perspective of behavioral change. In: GROSSI, S. A. A.; PASCALI, P. M. **Cuidados de enfermagem em Diabetes Mellitus**.

Sao Paulo: Brazilian Diabetes Society/Nursing Department of the Brazilian Diabetes Society, 2009.

GUYTON, A. C; HALL, J. E. **Treatise on medical physiology**. 12th ed. Rio de Janeiro: Guanabara Koogan, 2012.

OKOSHI, K. et al. Diabetic cardiomyopathy. **Arquivos Brasileiros de Endocrinologia e Metabologia**, v. 51, n. 2, p. 160-167, 2007.

REZENDE, H. A.; COCCO, M. I. M. The use of phytotherapy in the daily life of a rural population. **Revista da Escola de Enfermagem USP**, v. 36, n. 3, p. 282288, 2002.

ROCHA, F. D. et al. Diabetes mellitus and oxidative stress: natural products as targets for new therapeutic models. **Revista Brasileira de Farmàcia**, v. 87, n. 2, p. 49-54, 2006.

RUDGE, M. V. C. et al. Maternal daily hyperglycemia diagnosed by glycemic profile: a maternal and perinatal public health problem. **Revista Brasileira de Ginecologia e Obstetricia**, v. 27, n. 11, p. 691-697, 2005.

SACHS, A. Diabetes Mellitus. In: CUPPARI, L. **Guias de Medicina Ambulatorial e Hospitalar. Clinical Nutrition in Adults.** 2nd ed. Sao Paulo: Manole**.** UNIFESP, ch. 9, p. 171-188, 2002.

SANTOS, H. H. **Manual pràtico para elaboração de projetos, monografias, dissertaçôes e teses na área de saù**. 2a ed. Joao Pessoa: Ed. UFPB, 2004.

SARTORELLI, D. S.; FRANCO, L. J.; CARDOSO, M. A. Nutritional intervention and primary prevention of type 2 diabetes mellitus: a systematic review. **Caderno de Saùde Pùblica**, Rio de Janeiro, v. 22, n. 1, p. 7-18, 2006.

SARTORI, M. S. et al. Contribution of post-breakfast glycemia to glycemic control in patients with type 2 diabetes mellitus. **Arquivos Brasileiros de Endocrinologia e Metabologia**, v. 50, n. 1, p. 53-59, 2006.

SBD. BRAZILIAN DIABETES SOCIETY. **SBD Guidelines**. Sao Paulo: AC Farmacêutica Ltda, 2013.

SECOLI, R. S. Drug interactions: foundations for clinical nursing practice. **Revista da Escola de Enfermagem USP**, v. 35, n. 1, p. 28-34, 2001.

SEMGUPTA, A.; GHOSH, S.; BHATTACHARJEE, S. Allium vegetables in cancer prevention an overview. **Asian Pacific Journal of Cancer Prevention**, v. 5, n. 3, p. 237-45, 2004.

SILVA, K. L.; CECHINEL FILHO, V. Plants of the genus bauhinia: chemical composition and pharmacological potential. **Quimica Nova**, v. 25, n. 3, p. 449-454, 2002.

SILVA, J. P. A. et al. Medicinal plants used by patients with Type 2 Diabetes Mellitus for probable glycemic control in the Municipality of Jequié-BA.

Revista Saùde.Com, v. 4, n. 1, p. 10-18, 2008.

SPETHMANN, C. N. **Medicina Alternativa de A a Z**. Sao Paulo: Natureza, 2004.

ZAPAROLLI, M. R. et al. Functional foods in the management of diabetes mellitus.

Revista Ciência & Saùde, v. 6, n. 1, p. 12-17, 2013.

CHAPTER 6

SICKENING AND ANTI-INFLAMMATORY ACTIVITY OF *BARBATIMÂO* (STRYPHNODENDRON ADSTRINGENS): *A REVIEW*

Josilene Ferreira Barbosa[1]

Moises Kauan da Silva Félix[1]

Rosemary Lucena Rocha[1]

Maria das Graças Silva

1. Nursing undergraduates at Santa Emilia de Rodat College;

2. Master's Degree in Natural and Synthetic Bioactive Products, Federal University of Paraiba.

ABSTRACT: The use of medicinal plants is becoming more and more common among the general population, a fact that is based on popular belief and lately research has proven their efficacy, as well as phytotherapeutic medicines, which are affordable for the majority of the population. Among so many plants, *Stryphnodendron adstringens* stands out, better known as barbatimâo, barba-de-timâo, chorâozinho-roxo, barca da virgindade, uabatimô, abaramotemo, barca-da-mocidade, ibatimô, paricarana, faveiro and enche-cangalha, very common in the Brazilian cerrado. The bark of the stem is the part most commonly used as an anti-inflammatory, which is why it stands out for its medicinal properties. Studies show that the aqueous extract of barbatimâo bark has a significant healing effect on wounds, as well as anti-inflammatory, analgesic and gastric mucosa-protective activity. This research highlights the healing and anti-inflammatory activities of this plant, demonstrating its importance in folk medicine. This is an exploratory study in which a review was carried out of bibliographical sources such as scientific articles, printed books on the subject and the databases Google Scholar and Scielo. Barbatim has several uses in traditional medicine in the treatment of bleeding, inflammation, infections, ulcers, vaginal bleeding and gonorrhea. It also contains flavonoids, alkaloids, terpenes, steroids, protease inhibitors and tannins. Therefore, we can conclude that tannins are the components most present in barbatim, and these compounds have been associated with antimicrobial and anti-inflammatory effects, acting to heal wounds and burns by forming a protective layer on the mucosa or damaged tissue, through the tannin-protein complex and/or polysaccharides. The Ministry of Health, through the National Medicinal Plants Policy and the National Integrative and Complementary Practices Policy, has included Barbatimâo (*Stryphnodendron adstringens)* as part of the National List of Essential Medicines (RENAME) as a herbal medicine with proven healing action.

Keywords: Barbatimao. Healing. Anti-inflammatory.

1 INTRODUCTION

Around 80% of the population in developing countries make use of traditional medicine and use medicinal plants as an alternative in the treatment of various illnesses, which are then used to extract substances and used in medicine (FARNSWORTH; SOERJATO, 1985).

According to Rizzini and Mors (1995), many medicinal plants that are popularly used are found in the Brazilian cerrado, and there is already scientific evidence of their efficacy, which is already used by pharmaceutical laboratories where the substances used in medicines are extracted. Among them is barbatimao.

The barbatimao is a deciduous tree (a plant that loses its leaves during the dry season), with an elongated crown, 4 to 5 m high, with a twisted trunk, native to the cerrados of the Southeast and Midwest. The fruits are cylindrical, indehiscent pods, 6 to 9 cm long, with a large number of brown seeds, which bloom in January (LORENZI; MATOS, 2002).

Stryphnodendron adstringens is popularly known as barbatimao, barba-de-timao, choraozinho-roxo, casca da virgindade, uabatimô, abaramotemo, casca-da-mocidade, ibatimô, paricarana, faveiro and enche-cangalha (MEIRA et al., 2013).

Popularly, the bark of the stem is the part used as an anti-inflammatory and healing agent, for example: used to heal ulcers, gynecological diseases, as well as being known as the bark of virginity, because of its astringent properties (LORENZI; MATOS, 2002).

Barbatimao is used in traditional medicine to treat bleeding, inflammation, infections, ulcers, vaginal bleeding and gonorrhea. It also contains flavonoids, alkaloids, terpenes, steroids, protease inhibitors and tannins (LORENZI, 2000; CAMARGO, 1985; VASCONCELOS et al., 2004).

Therefore, the use of barbatim as a herbal alternative to other conventional medicines is justified by the fact that it has high healing power and anti-inflammatory activity. Another important factor in choosing this plant is the results already obtained through user reports, as well as the proof provided by various scientific studies, so it is necessary to add knowledge to the studies that are already available.

What is the importance of the healing and anti-inflammatory therapeutic actions found in barbatim (*Stryphnodendron adstringens*)?

In general, the population relies on popular knowledge passed down from parents to children, but scientific studies proving its efficacy will make it safer to use this valuable medicinal plant.

When researching the subject, it was observed that even with scientific advances in the study of *Stryphnodendron adstringens*, it is used on a daily basis, based on information passed down through the generations. Therefore, it is necessary to publicize the importance of a study that highlights the healing and anti-inflammatory activities of this plant, demonstrating its importance for folk medicine.

To clarify the rational use of *Stryphnodendron adstringens* as a healing and anti-inflammatory agent, to show the importance of barbatim due to its high therapeutic potential and to demonstrate how the healing and anti-inflammatory effects of this plant evolve.

2 MATERIAL AND METHODS

This is an exploratory type of research in terms of its objectives. The main purpose of exploratory research is to develop, clarify and modify concepts and ideas, with a view to formulating more precise problems or researchable hypotheses for further study (GIL, 2011).

As for the collection procedures, bibliographical research was used to compose the work, looking for information in studies already carried out. According to Gil (2011), bibliographical research is carried out using material that has already been prepared, consisting mainly of books and scientific articles.

A review was carried out of bibliographic sources such as scientific articles, printed books, magazines and the databases Google Scholar and Scielo.

A total of 25 articles related to the topic were found, of which 21 were selected, considering articles in Portuguese that dealt with the topic in question and as exclusion criteria, articles that were not linked to the proposed objectives were discarded, using as descriptors: barbatim, *Stryphnodendron adstringens*, healing and wounds.

3 RESULTS AND DISCUSSION

Stryphnodendron adstringens (Mar.) is a medicinal plant that contains tannins in its bark, as well as alkaloids, starch, flavonoids, proanthocyanidins, resinous and mucilaginous substances, dyes and saponins. Tannins are water-soluble phenolic substances and form water-insoluble complexes with alkaloids, gelatins and other substances. There are three general properties of tannins that are responsible for most of their pharmacological activities: the formation of complexes with metal ions, antioxidant and free radical scavenging activity and the ability to form complexes with other molecules such as proteins and polysaccharides (PEREIRA; MORENO; CARVALHO, 2013).

Tannins are the most common components of barbatim, and these compounds have been associated with antimicrobial effects. As an anti-inflammatory agent, they act to heal wounds and burns by forming a protective layer on the mucosa or injured tissue, through the tannin-protein complex and/or polysaccharides (MELLO, 1998).

Stryphnodendron adstringens (Mar.), popularly known as barbatimao, is a medicinal plant with great scientifically proven therapeutic value. This plant is promising for the development of a herbal medicine, but further studies and research are needed to validate this pharmacological potential (PEREIRA; MORENO; CARVALHO, 2013).

The importance of using herbal medicine as an alternative in the treatment of lesions is due to the fact that traditional antimicrobial agents no longer produce satisfactory results, in the view of Norton (2000), but under the recommendation of the WHO (1980), new technologies within the reach of the community should be used, with social security and economic sustainability. For many communities where access to conventional medicine is still scarce, the use of medicinal plants has become the only alternative treatment, even if there is no scientific proof, medicinal plants are used and this tradition is part of popular knowledge, passing on the knowledge to future generations (SILVA et al., 2010).

The Ministry of Health has been encouraging the use of medicinal plants as a complementary alternative; it has therefore been implementing the National Policy on Medicinal Plants and Phytotherapics (BRASIL, 2010). And in a list of 66 plants, 08 of which are cited as healing, *Stryphnodendron adstringens* (barbatimao) stands out, whose bark extract is the part of the plant most used in folk medicine because it contains a high concentration of tannins as its main active ingredient, around 20% (SILVA et al., 2010).

The commercial exploitation of barbatimao is purely extractive and is aimed at extracting tannins from the bark for use in folk medicine and for tanning animal hides. Tannins precipitate proteins and can combine with them to make them resistant. They are used to treat burns and skin abrasions. Studies show that the aqueous extract of barbatim bark has a significant healing effect on wounds and also has anti-inflammatory, analgesic and gastric mucosa-protective activity (PEREIRA; MORENO; CARVALHO, 2013).

In the view of Passaretti et al. (2016), when it comes to injuries, regardless of their origin and location on the human skin, what is expected is healing in the shortest possible time. Therefore, he defines wounds as "the loss of continuity of the integument, represented not only by the rupture of the skin and subcutaneous cellular tissue, but also by muscles, tendons and bones".

According to Minatel et al. (2010), condensed tannins stimulate the healing process as they bind to the proteins of injured tissues, creating a protective layer that insulates the wound site, reducing permeability and exudation and promoting tissue repair.

The extract obtained from the bark of *Stryphnodendron adstringens* shows antimicrobial activity against *Pseudonomas aeruginosas*, *Staphylococcus aereus* and *Bacillus subtilis*, as well as anti-inflammatory activity (SOUZA et al., 2007).

Clinical studies by Piriz et al. (2014) showed that there have been great advances in the use of medicinal plants as an alternative, especially barbatim (*Stryphnodendron adstringens).* This study was carried out with 27 patients over six months, who used barbatim extract to evaluate its effectiveness in healing decubitus ulcers, all of which obtained 100% satisfactory results.

Studies were also carried out by Pereira, Moreno and Carvalho (2013), in mice with the intention of evaluating the healing activity of barbatim, in skin wounds treated with typical daily use of 0.1 ml of aqueous barbatim solution did not show any purulent formation until the 14th day, but with the appearance of pus the use of the solution was continued and on the 19th day the epithelial tissue was restored.

According to Soares et al. (2008), studies have shown anti-inflammatory activity when using plates containing bacteria: *Enterococcus faecalis*, *Streptococcus salivarius*, *Streptococcus sanguinis*, *Streptococcus mitis*, *Streptococcus mutans*, *Streptococcus sobrinus* and *Lactobacillus casei*. Using microdilution techniques, the concentration of barbatimao extract varied between 50 and 400mg/ml. They were observed for 24 hours and bacterial inhibition was assessed.

4 CONCLUSIONS

It was then concluded that tannins are the most present components of barbatimao, and these compounds have been associated with antimicrobial and anti-inflammatory effects, acting to heal wounds and burns by forming a protective layer on the mucosa or injured tissue, through the tannin-protein complex and/or polysaccharides.

The Ministry of Health, through the National Medicinal Plants Policy and the National Integrative and Complementary Practices Policy, has included Barbatimao (*Stryphnodendron adstringens*) in the list of 66 medicinal plants that can be used and distributed by health services, thus integrating the RENAME (National List of Essential Medicines) as a herbal medicine with proven healing action.

REFERENCES

BRAZIL. Ministry of Health. National Health Surveillance Agency.

Resolution - RDC No. 10 of March 9, 2010. Provides for the notification of plant drugs. Brasilia, Ministry of Health, 2010.

CAMARGO, M. T. L. A. **Medicina popular:** aspectos metodológicos para pesquisa, garrafada, objeto de pesquisa, componentes medicinais de origem vegetal, animal e mineral. Sao Paulo: ALMED, 1985. 130p.

FARSNWORTH, N. R.; SOERJATO, D. D. Potential consequence of plant extinction in the United States on the current and future availlability of prescription drugs. **Economic Botany**, v. 39, p. 231-240, 1985.

GIL, A. C. **Métodos e técnicas de pesquisa social**. 5ª ed. Sao Paulo: Atlas, 2011.

LORENZI, H. **Arvores Brasileiras:** manual de identificaçâo e cultivo de plantas arbóreas do Brasil. 3rd ed. Nova Odessa: Instituto Plantarum, v. 1, 2000.

LORENZI, H.; MATOS, F. J. A. **Plantas Medicinais do Brasil Nativas e Exóticas**. Sao Paulo: Instituto Plantarum, 2002.

MEIRA, M. R. et al. Barbatimao: ecology, tannin production and socioeconomic potential in the northern region of Minas Gerais. **Enciclopédia Biosfera**, v. 9, n. 16, p. 466-94, 2013.

MELLO, J. C. Featured Plants: Barbatimao (Cortex). **Revista Racine**, v. 46, p. 42-43, 1998.

MINATEL, D. G. et al. Clinical study of the efficacy of ointment containing barbatimao

(*Stryphnodendron adstringens*) Coville in the healing of decubitus ulcers. **Revista Brasileira de Medicina**, v. 67, n.7, p. 250, 256, 2010.

NORTON, S. A. Botanical heritage of dermatology. In: AVALOS, J.; MAIBACH, H.I. **Dermatologic Botany**. CRC Press LCC: Boca Raton, 2000.

WHO. WORLD HEALTH ORGANIZATION. Health for all strategies for the year 2000. **Pan American Sanitary Bureau**. Official Document, n. 173, 1980.

PASSARETTI, T. et al. Efficacy of the use of barbatim (*Stryphnodendron barbatiman*) in the healing process of injuries: a literature review.

ABCS Health Sciences, v. 41, n. 1, p. 51-54, 2016.

PEREIRA, C.; MORENO, C. S.; CARVALHO, C. Pharmacological uses of

Stryphnodendron adstringens (Mar.) Barbatimâo. **Revista Panorâmica On-Line**, v. 15, p. 127-137, 2013.

PIRIZ, M. A. et al. Medicinal plants in the wound healing process: a literature review. **Revista Brasileira de Plantas Medicinais**, v. 16, n. 3, p. 628636, 2014.

RIZZINI, C. T.; MORS, W. B. **Botânica Econômica Brasileira**. 2a ed. Rio de Janeiro: Âmbito Cultural, p. 248, 1995.

SILVA, L. A. F. et al. Popular use of barbatimâo. In: SILVA, L. A. F.; EURIDES, D.; PAULA, J. R.; LIMA, C. R. O.; MOURA, M. I. **Manual do barbatimâo**.

Goiânia: Kelps, 2010.

SOARES, S. P. et al. Antibacterial activity of the crude hydroalcoholic extract of Stryphnodendron Adstringens on dental caries microorganisms. **Revista Odonto Ciência**, v. 23, n. 2, p. 141-144, 2008.

SOUZA, T. M. et al. Evaluation of the antiseptic activity of a dry extract of *Stryphnodendron adstringens* (Mart.) Coville and a cosmetic preparation containing this extract. **Revista Brasileira de Farmacognosia**, v. 17, n.1, p. 71-75, 2007.

VASCONCELOS, M. C. A. et al. Evaluation of the biological activity of the seeds of Stryphnodendron obovatum Benth (Leguminosae). **Revista Brasileira de Farmacognosia**, v. 14, n.2, p. 121-127, 2004.

CHAPTER 7

THE BENEFITS OF GREEN TEA (*CAMELLIA SIMENSIS)* AND ITS ANTIOXIDANT ACTIVITY: A REVIEW

Efraim de Britto Gomes Filho[1]

Maria das Graças Silva[2]

1. Graduating in Nursing from Santa Emilia de Rodat College;

2. Master's Degree in Natural and Synthetic Bioactive Products, Federal University of Paraiba.

SUMMARY: Antioxidants are a group of heterogeneous substances made up of vitamins, minerals, natural pigments and other natural components and enzymes that block the damaging effects of free radicals. They are obtained from food and are mostly found in vegetables, which explains part of the healthy effects that fruit, vegetables and whole grains have on the body. The human body naturally produces substances called free radicals, which can be defined as highly reactive atoms or molecules that contain an odd number of electrons in their last electronic layer, formed during routine processes in the body such as breathing and digesting food. Phytotherapy offers alternatives to traditional therapies, through teas, spices and other presentations aimed at improving the quality of health and the functional capacity of organs and systems. Green tea is rich in polyphenols or flavonoids, substances that have an antioxidant action superior to any other known natural antioxidant. Therefore, the aim of this study was to present the benefits of green tea and its antioxidant activity. This study is a bibliographical review, exploratory in its objectives and qualitative in nature. Flavonoids (catechins) are capable of promoting a reduction in body weight and fat, helping to prevent and treat obesity, dyslipidemia, diabetes, cardiovascular disorders, preventing the cellular alterations that cause tumours, neutralizing free radicals and fighting ageing. Daily consumption of this tea, combined with a healthy diet and regular physical activity, is excellent for the body's health. Studies have shown that the catechins present in green tea have therapeutic antioxidant properties, establishing a link with the prevention of ageing and the promotion of various beneficial effects on human health.

Keywords: Green tea. Antioxidant. Herbal medicine. Free radicals.

1 INTRODUCTION

Antioxidants can be defined as substances capable of slowing down or inhibiting the oxidation of oxidizable substrates, which can be enzymatic or non-enzymatic, such as: α-tocopherol (vitamin E), β-carotene, ascorbate (vitamin C) and phenolic compounds (flavonoids). The consumption of natural antioxidants, such as the phenolic compounds present in most plants, inhibits the formation of free radicals, also known as reactive substances (MORAIS et al., 2009).

The human body naturally produces substances called free radicals, which can be defined as highly reactive atoms or molecules that contain an odd number of electrons in their last electronic layer, formed in routine body processes such as respiration and food digestion (NEVES et al., 2014).

Oxidation is indispensable for aerobic life and free radicals are therefore produced naturally. These molecules generated in vivo are involved in energy production, phagocytosis, cell growth regulation, intercellular signaling and the synthesis of important biological substances (BARREIROS; DAVID; DAVID, 2006).

The excess of free radicals in the body is combated by antioxidants which are produced by the body or absorbed through the diet. When there is an imbalance between the production of free radicals and the antioxidant defense mechanisms, what is known as oxidative stress occurs (OLIVEIRA et al., 2011).

Green tea has been known in China for over 4,000 years as a powerful ally for good health. It is rich in polyphenols or flavonoids, substances that have an antioxidant (anti-free radical) action superior to any other known natural antioxidant (SIMÔES et al., 2004). Phytotherapy offers alternatives to traditional therapies, through teas, spices and other presentations, with the aim of improving the quality of health and the functional capacity of organs and systems. Green tea is made from the infusion of the herb *Camellia sinensis* and is called "green" because the leaves of the herb undergo little oxidation during processing (MACHADO, 2012).

Camellia sinesis can also be called Indian tea, and its leaves contain around 30% of the total composition of polyphenolic compounds, mainly epicatechins, whose main therapeutic property is antioxidant (SIMÔES et al., 2004). Flavonoids (catechins) are capable of promoting a reduction in body weight and fat, helping to prevent and treat obesity, dyslipidemia, diabetes, cardiovascular disorders, preventing the cellular alterations that cause tumors, neutralizing free radicals and fighting aging. Green tea contains catechins such as epicatechins (EC), epigallocatechins (ECG) and epigallocatechin gallate (EGCG), the latter being more abundant in green tea and are constituents related to the prevention of ageing (MACHADO, 2012).

Green tea has high concentrations of carotenes and vitamins C and E, which rejuvenate the body. It is also rich in manganese, potassium, folic acid and vitamins C, K, B1 and B2, as well as being a good source of tannins. Daily consumption of this tea, combined with a healthy diet and regular physical activity, is excellent for the body's health (SIMÔES et al., 2004).

The topic was chosen to clarify the importance of green tea and its antioxidant action. The following question arises: What is the antioxidant activity of green tea and what are its benefits? The aim of this study was therefore to present the benefits of green tea and its antioxidant activity, as well as to clarify the benefits of this tea, report on the importance of antioxidants, identify the effects of free radicals and characterize the antioxidant function of green tea.

2 MATERIAL AND METHODS

This study consisted of a bibliographical review, exploratory in its objectives and qualitative in nature. To this end, 20 scientific articles were searched using the electronic databases: Google Scholar, Scielo, from which 18 articles were obtained. The inclusion criteria were national journals that were linked to the proposed theme, and the exclusion criteria were all articles that were not directly related to the theme. The following indexed terms were used for the search: green tea, antioxidant, phytotherapy and free radicals.

According to Gil (2011), a bibliographic review is the collection of data from studies that have already been published and that have relevance to the problem under study, consisting not only of what has already been published, but also of a discussion of ideas, foundations, problems, suggestions, among others, so that it is clear that the articles researched have actually been examined, criticized and summarized.

In order to achieve the objectives, the bibliographical research was carried out in the following stages: choice of topic, preliminary bibliographical survey, formulation of the problem, elaboration of the problem, elaboration of the provisional plan of the subject, searches for sources, reading of the material, logical organization of the subject and writing of the text, to conclude the monograph.

3 Results and discussion

Since ancient times, plants have been used as medicines to prevent, treat and cure disorders, dysfunctions or diseases in humans and animals. Green tea is consumed mainly in Asian countries, where its meaning goes beyond a simple drink, being synonymous with prosperity, harmony, beauty and its consumption becomes a ritual of great social and cultural importance (RATES, 2001 apud CLARKE; RATES; BRIDI, 2007).

About a century ago, the tea drink arrived in Brazil in the hands of Chinese immigrants, who introduced the secrets of planting, burning, handling and standardizing the product and with this it spread to the states of Paranà, Sao Paulo, Rio de Janeiro and Minas Gerais. Brazil has a great plant biodiversity and at least half of the plant species may possess some therapeutic property. There are hundreds of types of tea that appeal to millions of people around the world and are an additional resource in the treatment of illnesses, sometimes dispensing with pharmacies. The benefits of teas are innumerable, but they should not be consumed in excess, as they also have adverse effects (ROHMER, 2002).

Tea in general, one of the most widely consumed beverages in the world, is one of the richest sources of flavonoids, antioxidant substances that act at different levels to protect the body and help neutralize free radicals, preventing their formation and which are responsible for premature cellular ageing (ROHMER, 2002; MATSUBARA; RODRIGUEZ-AMAYA, 2006).

Tea made from the leaves of the *Camellia sinensis* plant is, after water, the most consumed non-alcoholic drink in the world. For centuries, tea has been considered a healthy drink by the Orientals and has been used in China for approximately 3,000 years, which is its main producer. *Camellia sinensis* is widely cultivated in South Asia, including China, India, Japan, Thailand, Sri Lanka and Indonesia (RIETVELD; WISEMAN, 2003; TANAKA; KOUNO, 2003).

Green tea, which used to be consumed as a medicine, has become popular due to its organoleptic characteristics, flavor and aroma. Its flavonoid and catechin components have a range of biological activities: chemoprotective, thermogenic, anti-inflammatory, anticarcinogenic, potent antioxidants, free radical scavengers, metal chelators (which would reduce their absorption) and lipoperoxidation inhibitors (SCHMITZ et al., 2005).

It is a non-fermented drink with a very varied chemical composition, although its beneficial effects are associated with catechins, it also contains water, protein, carbohydrates, vitamins (mainly vitamins C and K), mineral salts, methylxanthines, which are responsible for adverse effects and drug interactions and, being stimulants of the central nervous system, its main representatives are caffeine, theophylline and theobromine, it also contains tannin and fluorine. Its composition varies according to the species, time of year, age of the leaves, climate and agronomic practices (HERNANDEZ-FIGUEROA; RODRIGUEZ-RODRIGUEZ; SANCHEZ-MUNIZ, 2004).

Caffeine is considered a stimulant drug, it has an effect on mental and behavioral function, is a diuretic, produces excitement, euphoria, reduces feelings of fatigue, increases motor activity and can negatively affect the quality of sleep. It is present in green tea in smaller quantities than is found in coffee, with a cup of tea containing around 6% caffeine, while a cup of coffee contains up to 25% (VALENZUELA, 2004). Teas are rich in biologically active compounds which, when added to the diet, trigger metabolic or physiological processes: flavonoids, catechins, polyphenols and alkaloids which contribute to the prevention and treatment of various diseases. Green tea has been widely used due to the presence of these compounds, its leaf contains around 30% phenolic compounds, which contribute to the taste, aroma and color of vegetables in general (SCHMITZ et al., 2005).

The beneficial effects of green tea have also been attributed to catechins, one of the classes of flavonoids, especially epigallocatechin gallate (EGCG), which have been making headlines since around the 80s. EGCG is also often referred to as the main ingredient in green tea, which is considered, however, to be too short. Focusing on ECGC, this is also likely to change because the catechin substances can be extracted as a green tea extract and used as a dietary supplement, which many studies have shown to have positive effects on various diseases as well as prevention. The greatest health benefit of green tea lies in the interaction of all the active ingredients and in high-quality preparation (FARIA et al., 2006).

4 CONCLUSIONS

Studies have shown that *Camellia simensis* has flavonoids of the catechin type that can help reduce body weight, prevent and treat obesity, dyslipidemia, diabetes, cardiovascular disorders, prevent the cellular changes that cause tumors, and has antioxidant therapeutic properties, neutralizing free radicals and fighting aging, thus promoting various benefits to human health.

REFERENCES

BARREIROS, A. L.; DAVID, J. M.; DAVID, J. P. Oxidative stress:

relationship between the generation of reactive species and the body's defense. **Quimica Nova**, v. 29, n. 1, p. 113-123, 2006.

CLARKE, J. H. R.; RATES, S. M. K.; BRIDI, R. A warning about the use of products of plant origin in pregnancy. **Revista Informa**, v. 19, n. 1/2, p. 41-48, 2007.

FARIA, F. et al. Consumption of *Camellia sinensis* in a population of oriental origin and incidence of chronic diseases. **Revista de Nutriçâo**, Campinas, v. 19, n. 2, p. 275279, 2006.

GIL, A. C. **Métodos e técnicas de pesquisa social.** 5ª ed. Sao Paulo: Atlas, 2011.

HERNANDEZ-FIGUEIROA, T. T.; RODRIGUEZ-RODRIGUEZ, E.; SANCHEZ- MUNIZ, F. J. Green tea, a good choice for the prevention of cardiovascular diseases. **Archivos Latino Americanos de Nutrición**, v. 54, n. 4, p. 380394, 2004.

MACHADO, F. C. S. **The effect of *Camellia sinensis* (green tea) on antioxidant activity and diseases**. 2012. 32f. Monograph. Faculty of Medical Sciences - PB. Joao Pessoa, 2012.

MATSUBARA, S.; RODRIGUEZ-AMAYA, D. B. Contents of catechins and theoflavins in teas marketed in Brazil. **Revista Ciência Tecnologia Alimentaçâo**, v. 26, n. 2, p. 401-407, 2006.

MORAIS, S. M. et al. Antioxidant action of teas and condiments widely consumed in Brazil. **Revista Brasileira de Farmacognosia**. v. 19, n. 1, p. 315-320, 2009.

NEVES, G. Y. S. et al. Evaluation of the consumption of antioxidant-rich foods and knowledge of free radicals by FAFIMAN Biological Sciences and Nursing students. **Revista Diàlogo & Saberes**, v.10, n.1, p. 47-62, 2014.

OLIVEIRA, D. S. et al. Vitamin C, carotenoids, total phenolics and antioxidant activity of guava, mango and papaya from Ceasa in the State of Minas Gerais. **Acta Scientiarum**, v. 33, n. 1, p. 89-98, 2011.

RHOMER, F. **The Book of Tea**. Trad. M. Dadonas. Sao Paulo: Aquariana, 2002.

RIETVELD, A.; WISEMAN, S. Antioxidant effects of tea: evidence from human clinical trials. **Journal of Nutrition**, v. 133, p. 3275-84, 2003.

SCHIMITZ, W. et al. Green tea and its actions as a chemoprotector. **Semina: Ciências**

Biológicas e da Saùde, v. 26, n. 2, p. 119-130, 2005.

SIMÔES, C. M. O. et al. **Farmacognosia - Da Planta ao Medicamento**. 5ª ed. Editora da UFRGS, Porto Alegre, 2004.

TANAKA, T.; KOUNO, I. Oxidation of tea catechins: chemical structures and reaction mechanism. **Food Science and Technology Research**, v. 9, p. 128-33, 2003.

VALENZUELA, A. B. Tea consumption and health: characteristics and beneficial properties of this ancient drink. **Revista Chilena de Nutrición**, v. 31, n. 2, p. 72-82, 2004.

CHAPTER 8

THE USE OF HERBAL MEDICINES IN THE TREATMENT OF OBESITY: A REVIEW

Ruanniere de Oliveira Silva[1]

Larissa de Fàtima Romao da Silva[1]

Bruno Rafael Virginio de Sousa[2]

Yohanna de Oliveira[3]

1. Undergraduate student in Nutrition at the Federal University of Paraiba;

2. Postgraduate student in Sports Nutrition, Faculdades Integradas de Patos (FIP);

3. Master's student in Nutritional Sciences, Federal University of Paraiba.

ABSTRACT: Obesity is a serious health problem all over the world, leading to various pathophysiological diseases such as hyperlipidemia, diabetes mellitus and congestive heart disease; however, there are few studies on the subject. The aim of this study was therefore to present current approaches to the treatment of obesity from the point of view of the use of herbal medicines. It consisted of a bibliographical review through searches in the Sciencedirect, Pubmed, Web of Science and CAPES journals, over a 7-year period, in English, and the terms indexed were herbal medicines, obesity, nutrition. Increased fat deposition may be the result of the predominant consumption of hyperlipidemic diets. The primary treatment for obesity is diet and exercise. To complement this, or in case of failure, anti-obesity drugs can be administered to reduce appetite or inhibit fat absorption. The lack of availability of drugs for their treatment is also a major concern, since fat-reducing drugs can also have implications for the liver, heart and spleen. Natural products identified from traditional medicinal plants have always presented an innovative opportunity for the development of new therapeutic agents. It was concluded that herbal medicines are important aids in the prevention of obesity, which is a multifactorial metabolic disease, as well as being inexpensive.

Keywords: Herbal medicines. Obesity. Nutrition.

1 INTRODUCTION

Obesity is a serious health problem worldwide, leading to various pathophysiological diseases such as hyperlipidemia, diabetes mellitus and congestive heart disease. Among the many factors that contribute to its etiology are a sedentary lifestyle, physical inactivity, endocrine disorders, physiological and psychological factors, smoking and late pregnancy, certain medications that increase body weight, mental illness and the consumption of high-calorie foods (D'MELLO; DARJI; SHETGIRI, 2011).

According to the aforementioned authors, obesity increases the mechanical and metabolic load on the myocardium, thus increasing the organ's oxygen consumption. Increased fat deposition may be the result of the predominant consumption of hyperlipidemic diets, the primary treatment for obesity being diet together with physical activity.

Drug treatments should always be combined with diet and exercise and should be targeted at obese patients who have not responded to conventional treatment. However, many drugs for the treatment of obesity (amphetamines, fenfluramine derivatives, rimonabant and others) have been withdrawn from the market due to their unfavorable risk-benefit ratio. The long-term effectiveness of appetite suppressants is questionable. Even if they lead to weight loss at the start of treatment, the weight reduction attributable to anorexigens (i.e. the weight loss that exceeds that achieved with diet and exercise alone) is generally modest, and partial weight regain occurs when they are used for longer than a year. In almost all cases, the weight loss achieved with appetite suppressants is reversed when the drug is stopped (PAUMGARTTEN, 2011).

The search for treatments with phytotherapics and medicinal plants has gained prominence in recent years, especially with a focus on obesity, but there is little scientific evidence about it. Corrêa, Santos and Ribeiro (2012) report that many authors emphasize the need for health professionals to be better qualified to handle herbal medicines.

Interest in medicines derived from medicinal plants has increased significantly around the world. This interest is especially observed in developed countries, mainly in some European countries and in the United States. It is estimated that the global market for this class of drugs has reached 20 billion dollars annually. In particular, plant-derived compounds are currently used in modern therapy, as well as playing an important role in the synthesis of some more complex molecules (DUTRA et al., 2016).

Manenti (2010) states that due to the dangerous side effects and high cost of drugs traditionally used to treat obesity, the potential of natural products to treat the disease is still being investigated and could be a viable alternative for the future development of effective and safe anti-obesity drugs.

Evidence has shown that many natural products can help treat obesity by acting on five different mechanisms described by Yun (2010), such as substances that (1) decrease lipid absorption, (2) decrease carbohydrate absorption, (3) increase energy expenditure, (4) decrease the differentiation and proliferation of preadipocytes, (5) decrease lipogenesis and increase lipolysis.

Among the products used, there are numerous medicinal plants, herbal medicines and/or nutraceuticals, used as adjuncts in the treatment of obesity because they have chemical components such as flavonoids, alkaloids, terpenoids, among others that favor weight loss, mainly with hypolipidemic, hypocholesterolemic, antihyperglycemic, anti-hyperlipidemic and antioxidant activity (YUN, 2010).

Since there is a lot of information on the use of herbal medicines and they are not so well elucidated in the treatment of obesity, we were interested in carrying out this study in order to be able to select those that have a reliable result, thus contributing to clarifying the subject. With this in mind, the aim of this study was to present current approaches to the treatment of obesity using herbal medicines.

2 MATERIAL AND METHODS

This was a literature review involving the collection and analysis of various scientific articles on the chosen topic. For the bibliographic survey, data was searched in the electronic databases Sciencedirect, Pubmed, Web Of Science and Periódicos CAPES, over a 10-year period, using the index terms: herbal medicines, obesity, nutrition.

Of the 30 articles searched, 24 were selected. The inclusion criteria were articles in English and Portuguese, from 2006 to 2016, which covered the effects of herbal medicines and the benefits they provide for obesity prevention. The exclusion criteria were articles that did not belong to the 2006 to 2016 timeframe, articles that did not present the benefits caused by them and experimental studies.

3 RESULTS AND DISCUSSION

Phytotherapy, present in all human societies, has been used and documented for its valuable traditional and popular knowledge resulting from its rich ethnic and cultural diversity (CORRÊA; SANTOS; RIBEIRO, 2012). In recent decades, researchers have devoted significant efforts to understanding the physiological mechanisms involved in controlling appetite, hunger and satiety, and to obtaining effective products for the treatment and control of obesity, including those of natural origin (MANENTI, 2010).

The increase in demand for herbal medicines can be associated with a healthier and less harmful alternative to treatment and with public dissatisfaction related to the lack of access to industrialized medicines. Health professionals have started to encourage the revaluation of the use of herbal medicines, seeking to improve and produce them on an industrial scale, unlike the artisanal forms that characterized the initial stages of their use (TUROLLA; NASCIMENTO, 2006; ROSA;

CÂMARA; BÉRIA, 2011).

In the review study carried out by Manenti (2010), 59 plants were listed as being used to treat obesity. According to the author, the vast majority did not present validated studies attesting to safety or proof of the expected effects. Only 25 articles presented studies on human beings. The main physiological mechanisms described in the articles were: lipase inhibition, thermogenic action and appetite-suppressing or satiety-increasing action. Of the 59 medicinal plants cited, only 13 have been tested on humans: *Caralluma fimbriata*, *Garcinia cambogia*, *Camellia sinensis, Phaseolus vulgaris* (white beans), *Ilex paraguariensis* (yerba mate), *Citrus Aurantium*, *Hoodia gordonii*, *Capsicum annum* (pepper), *Coffea aràbica* (coffee), *Gymnema sylvestre*, *Pinus koraiensis* (Korean pine), *Cissus quadrangularis* and *Irvingia gabonensis* (African mango).

According to Weisheimer et al. (2015) in a review study, they found that most clinical studies have shown weight reduction through the use of herbal medicines, which act through different mechanisms of action. The main herbal medicines that were discussed and showed positive results in the treatment of obesity were: *Camelia sinensis* (green tea), which has a mainly thermogenic effect, *Cynara scolymus* (artichoke), which acts significantly in weight reduction when associated with physical activity, and *Phaseolus vulgaris* (white beans), which acts by reducing the absorption of carbohydrates in the intestine.

Green tea originated in China and is grown and consumed in more than 160 countries, especially in Asia (KUMUDAVALLY et al., 2008). *Camellia sinensis* teas have different popular names, such as green tea, black tea, white tea and red tea. This classification is due to the different ways in which the leaves are harvested and processed. Of the four types of tea, green tea is the richest in compounds with thermogenic activities (CHENG, 2006).

It has various biological activities, including antioxidant and anti-obesity, due to its thermogenic effect, as well as being effective in reducing cholesterol levels, immunostimulatory, antimicrobial and antioxidant activities, helping to prevent chronic degenerative diseases such as cancer and cardiovascular diseases (LUO; CANIGGIA; POST, 2014).

Cynara scolymus L., popularly known as artichoke, belongs to the Astreaceae family. It is a plant that originated in North Africa and grows in Brazil in regions with a subtropical climate, with temperatures between 5°C and 30°C (SILVA, 2013). Pancreatic lipase inhibition has been identified as one of the most widely studied mechanisms for determining the potential of natural products as anti-obesity agents. The artichoke (*Cynara scolymus* L.), in turn, has potential as an adjuvant in the treatment of obesity and dyslipidemia, since it inhibits the activity of the pancreatic lipase enzyme (SOUZA et al., 2012).

The consumption of legumes has also been associated with a reduction in the risk of developing chronic non-communicable diseases, including diabetes, cancer, obesity and cardiovascular diseases (SCHORODER, 2007; SIEVENPIPER et al., 2009; CAMPOS-VEJA et al., 2013). The common bean, with the scientific name *Phaseolus vulgaris*, is a legume considered to be a rich source of nutrients and has long been used in Brazil as a staple food for the population, both in rural and urban areas (RAMiREZ-CARDENAS; LEONEL; COSTA, 2008).

The explanation best elucidated in the literature for the treatment of obesity with the consumption of such food is that white beans prevent the breakdown of larger carbohydrates by blocking α-amylase, and consequently reduce postprandial glycemia, in addition to prolonging gastric emptying, thus contributing to increased satiety (CELLENO et al., 2007; PEREIRA et al., 2010; BARRETT; UDANI, 2011; HAYAT et al., 2014).

4 CONCLUSIONS

From the present study, it was concluded that there is information that needs to be better elucidated in the scientific literature on the use of herbal medicines in the treatment of obesity, where it has been shown that herbal medicines have a positive response to the treatment of the disease, acting as an adjunct, but the mechanisms by which this response occurs are not yet well explained.

Most studies report that this market has been growing in recent years, both because of the positive response to treatment and because of the ease of access and increase in the number of prescriptions by health professionals following the regulation of their use, but studies have shown that a large proportion of these herbal medicines are still not validated.

REFERENCES

BARRETT, M. L.; UDANI, J. K. A Proprietary Alphaamylase Inhibitor From White Bean (Phaseolus vulgaris): A Review of Clinical Studies on Weight Loss and Glycemic Control. **Nutrition Journal**, v. 17, p. 10-24, 2011.

CAMPOS-VEJA, R. et al. Common Beans and Their Non-Digestible Fraction: Cancer Inhibitory Activity-An Overview. **Foods**, v. 2, n. 3, p.374-392, 2013.

CELLENO, L. et al. A Dietary Supplement Containing Standardized Phaseolus vulgaris Extract Influences Body Composition of Overweight Men and Women. **International Journal of Medical Sciences**, v. 24, n. 4, p. 45-52, 2007.

CHENG, T. O. All teas are not created equal: the chinese green tea and cardiovascular health. **International Journal of Cardiology**, v. 108, n. 3, p. 301308, 2006.

CORRÊA, E. D. M.; SANTOS, J. M.; RIBEIRO, P. L. B. **Uso de Fitoteràpicos no Tratamento da Obesidade: Uma Revisâo Bibliogràfica**. Goiânia, 2012. 25p. Course Conclusion Work - Pontifical Catholic University of Goiás, 2012.

D'MELLO, P. M.; DARJI, K. K.; SHETGIRI, P. P. Evaluation of Antiobesity Activity of Various Plant Extracts. **Pharmacognosy Journal**, v. 3, n. 21, p. 56-59, 2011.

DUTRA, R. C. et al. Medicinal plants in Brazil: Pharmacological studies, drug discovery, challenges and perspectives. **Pharmacological Research,** v. 112, p. 429, 2016.

HAYAT, I. et al. Nutritional and Health Perspectives of Beans (Phaseolus vulgaris L.): an Overview. **Critical Reviews in Food Science and Nutrition**, v. 54, n. 5, p. 580-92, 2014.

KUMUDAVALLY, K. V. et al. Green tea - a potential preservative for extending the shelf life of fresh mutton at ambient temperature (25 ± 2 °C). **Food Chemistry**, v. 107, n. 1, p. 426-433, 2008.

LUO, D.; CANIGGIA, I.; POST, M. Hypoxia Inducible Regulation of Placental BOK Expression. **Biochemical Journal**, v. 461, n. 3, p. 391-402, 2014.

MANENTI, A. V. **Medicinal plants used in the treatment of obesity: A review**. Santa Catarina, 2010. 83p. Course Conclusion Paper (Graduation in Nutrition) - Universidade do Extremo Sul Catarinense - UNESC, 2010.

PAUMGARTTEN, F. J. R. Pharmacological treatment of obesity: the public health perspective. **Cadernos de Saùde Pùblica**, v. 27, n. 3, p. 404-405, 2011.

PEREIRA, L. L. S. et al. Precipitation of α-Amylase Inhibitor from White Beans: Evaluation of Methods. **Alimentos e Nutriçâo**, v. 21, n. 1, p. 15-20, 2010.

RAMiREZ-CARDENAS, L. A.; LEONEL, A. J.; COSTA, N. M. B. Effect of Domestic Processing on the Nutrient Content and Antinutritional Factors of Different Cultivars of Common Beans. **Ciência e Tecnologia de Alimentos**, v. 28, p. 200-213, 2008.

ROSA, C.; CÂMARA, S. G.; BÉRIA, J. U. Representations and intention to use phytotherapy in primary health care. **Ciência & Saùde Coletiva**, v. 16, n. 1, p. 311-318, 2011.

SCHRODER, H. J. Protective Mechanism of the Mediterranean Diet in Obesity and Type 2 Diabetes. **The Journal of Nutritional Biochemistry**, v.18, n. 3, p.149-60, 2007.

SIEVENPIPER, J. L. et al. Effect of non-oil-seed Pulses on Glycaemic Control: a Systematic Review and Meta-analysis of Randomized Controlled Experimental Trials in People With and Without Diabetes. **Diabetologia**, v. 52, n. 8, p.1479-95, 2009.

SILVA, M. E. M. **Study of Medicinal Plants Popularly Used in the Treatment of Obesity in Ararangua - Santa Catarina**. 2013. 83p. Course Conclusion Work (Graduation in Biological Sciences) - Federal University of Santa Catarina - UFSC, 2013.

SOUZA, S. P. et al. Selection of Crude Extracts of Plants with Antiobesity Activity. **Revista Brasileira de Plantas Medicinais**, v. 14, n. 4, p. 643-648, 2012.

TUROLLA, M. S. R.; NASCIMENTO, E. S. Toxicological information on some herbal medicines used in Brazil. **Revista Brasileira de Ciências Farmacêuticas**, v. 42, n. 2, p. 289-306, 2006.

WEISHEIMER, N. et al. Phytotherapy as a Therapeutic Alternative in the Fight against Obesity. **Revista Ciência e Saùde Nova Esperança**, v. 13, n. 1, p. 103-111, 2015.

YUN, J. W. Possible Anti-obesity Therapeutics from Nature: A Review. **Phytochemistry**, v. 71, n. 14-15, p.1625-1641, 2010.

CHAPTER 9

THE RELATIONSHIP BETWEEN THE USE OF GREEN TEA AND ITS BENEFICIAL EFFECTS ON DYSLIPIDEMIA: A REVIEW OF THE LITERATURE

Larissa de Fàtima Romao da Silva[1]

Ruanniere de Oliveira Silva[1]

Bruno Rafael Virginio de Sousa[2]

Yohanna de Oliveira[3]

1. Undergraduate student in Nutrition at the Federal University of Paraiba;

2. Postgraduate student in Sports Nutrition, Faculdades Integradas de Patos (FIP);

3. Master's student in Nutritional Sciences, Federal University of Paraiba.

ABSTRACT: In recent years, due to the fast pace of life, stress and practicality have taken center stage in people's lives, and healthy eating has lost its place. The combination of these factors has led to an exorbitant number of people suffering from cardiovascular diseases, especially those with high levels of LDL and total cholesterol and low levels of HDL. This data is alarming and has led cardiac patients to look for healthier alternatives to help treat cardiovascular diseases. Among the nutritional strategies available, one of the most studied today is green tea, which is produced from the processing of the *Camellia sinensis* plant. Given the scientific evidence, the aim of this study was to present the potential beneficial effects of green tea on dyslipidemia, and consequently on cardiovascular health and improved quality of life. This is a bibliographical review, through searches in the Pubmed, Sciencedirect and Periódicos Capes databases, in English and Portuguese. It was observed that regular consumption of green tea was able to reduce glycerol, total cholesterol, LDL and triglycerides and there was an increase in HDL, especially in obese patients. Experimental studies have shown that tea consumption was able to significantly reduce body weight and weight gain. In addition, it was possible to observe a reduction in the weight of the liver, kidneys, muscles, perirenal, mesenteric, interscapular and visceral tissue. According to all the research analyzed, several indicators show scientifically-based arguments that highlight the importance of regular consumption and adequate amounts of green tea, so that it can provide its benefits for the cardiovascular health of the population affected by these problems, which have become the main cause of death for Brazilians of both sexes.

Keywords: Green tea. Dyslipidemia. Obesity. Polyphenols.

1 INTRODUCTION

Despite their reduction, cardiovascular diseases (CVD) have been and continue to be the leading cause of death in Brazil (SCHMIDT et al., 2011). In addition, CVDs are responsible for the highest cost of hospital admissions in the national health system (IBGE, 2009). In this context, recent studies have shown that the combined consumption of green and black tea leads to a significant reduction in mortality; however, only the consumption of green tea was related to a reduction in the risk of cardiovascular mortality. This complication was reduced by 5% for every cup of green tea (*Camellia sinensis*) consumed per day (TANG et al., 2015).

Camellia sinensis is a plant of Asian origin, belonging to the Theaceae family. From the processing of this plant, green tea, oolong (tea that has the oxidation process between green and black tea) and black tea are obtained, resulting from the differential fermentation of the leaves (SA; TURELLA; BETTEGA, 2007). To produce green tea, the polyphenol oxidase is inactivated and the dried leaves are subjected to dry heat, preserving their phenolic compounds (PIMENTEL; FRANCKI; GOLLÜCKE, 2005).

Green tea has been widely studied for its beneficial effects in human and animal studies, with the functional properties of tea being highlighted due to its polyphenolic compounds. The main catechins in green tea are epigallocatechin gallate (EGCG), epigallocatechin (EGC), epicatechin gallate (ECG), epicatechin (EC) and catechin (C). The most abundant and active catechin in green tea is EGCG (NAGLE; FERREIRA; ZHOU, 2006). Among the effects attributed to green tea catechins, beneficial effects have been reported, such as: anti-obesity, antioxidant, anti-hypertensive, anti-diabetic and anti-inflammatory (BOSE et al., 2008; PARK et al., 2011; BASU et al., 2013).

In this perspective, the consumption of catechins present in green tea in supplements of capsule or powder, has shown to have marked effects on the reduction of LDL cholesterol (ONAKPOYA et al., 2014; ZHENG et al., 2013). Catechins are antioxidants that prevent LDL oxidation both in vitro and in vivo in humans (SUZUKI-SUGIHARA et al., 2016). Tests have been carried out to evaluate the effect of green tea consumption on lipid parameters and the result was a significant reduction in serum concentrations, showing an effect on the lipid profile (ONAKPOYA et al., 2014; ZHENG et al., 2013; HOOPER et al., 2008).

In view of the scientific evidence, the aim of this study was to present the potential beneficial effects of green tea on dyslipidemia, and consequently on cardiovascular health and improved quality of life.

2 MATERIAL AND METHODS

This is a literature review involving the analysis of various scientific articles on the chosen topic. For the bibliographic survey, data was searched in the electronic databases Pubmed, Periódicos CAPES and Sciencedirect, using literature from the last 12 years, with the index terms: green tea, dyslipidemia, cardiovascular disease and cholesterol.

Of the 15 articles found, 7 were selected for this review. The inclusion criteria were articles in English and Portuguese, from 2000 to 2017, which covered the benefits of green tea consumption for improving the blood lipid profile and preventing cardiovascular diseases. The exclusion criteria were articles that did not belong to the time interval between 2000 and 2017 and articles that did not focus on the benefits of green tea for reducing serum cholesterol levels.

3 RESULTS AND DISCUSSION

To assess the effect of catechins on reducing body fat and the relationship between oxidized LDL and body fat variables, Nagao et al. (2005) evaluated the effects of consuming oolong tea, which contains large amounts of catechins. For 12 weeks, Japanese men drank a bottle of oolong tea a day. Compared to the control group, those who consumed green tea had a reduction in abdominal circumference, skinfolds and subcutaneous and total body fat, as well as a reduction in LDL levels.

Batista et al. (2009) carried out a double-blind cross-over study in which 38 patients with dyslipidemia were given capsules containing 250 mg of dry extract of green tea (*Camelia sinensis*) or placebo for 16 weeks. During the study, 5 participants dropped out, leaving 33 volunteers who completed the study. As a result, there was a variation in weight and BMI of around 1.7% between the groups. There was also a variation in serum cholesterol levels, especially in plasma LDL, thus demonstrating that green tea had a positive effect on body weight, BMI and LDL.

Another study carried out by Teixeira, Zancanaro and Santos (2012) showed a positive reduction in cholesterol and BMI when green tea was consumed, but with regard to plasma triglyceride concentrations, there was no significant effect of the treatment, perhaps because some volunteers did not fast for 12 hours the day before the sample was taken, as was explained to them to avoid interference. This study showed that the compounds found in this herbal medicine, such as catechins, reduce cholesterol and triglyceride levels. Other components such as caffeine and polyphenols increase energy expenditure by oxidizing fats and reducing body weight.

Raederstorff et al. (2003) carried out a study using a high-cholesterol diet and supplementation with 0.25% (0.2g/kg body weight/day), 0.5% (0.4g/kg body weight/day) and 1.0% (0.7g/kg body weight/day) EGCG in wistar rats. After 4 weeks, the group receiving 1% epigallocatechin gallate showed significantly lower total cholesterol and LDL plasma levels compared to the control group. There was also a considerable reduction in the absorption of cholesterol in the intestine in the group supplemented with high doses of epigallocatechin gallate, i.e. 1.0% (0.7g/kg of weight/day). Yokozawa, Nakagawa and Kitani (2002) also showed significant results of green tea in inhibiting LDL oxidation and raising HDL in rats, which is different to the result found by Raederstorff et al. (2003), who did not identify significant increases in HDL.

Kao, Hiipakka and Liao (2000) studied the effects of epigallocatechin gallate on the endocrine system in adult rats of both sexes. Male rats were given 85mg of epigallocatechin gallate/kg body weight intraperitoneally for 7 days and showed a weight reduction of 30-41% compared to the control group. In females, approximately 92mg/kg of weight was administered, which induced weight loss of 10 and 29% compared to the initial body weight and the control group. In agreement, Murase et al. (2002) observed that supplementation with 0.2 and 0.5% green tea extract and a high-fat diet for a period of 11 months led to a considerably lower hepatic content of triglycerides when compared to the group that received only a high-fat diet.

In the review study carried out by Hernandez-Figueroa, Rodriguez-Rodriguez and Sanches-Muniz (2004), the authors concluded that the consumption of 7 cups of green tea a day would be a good recommendation for the prevention of cardiovascular diseases, when associated with a balanced diet and exercise.

4 CONCLUSIONS

In view of the studies available and the fact that cardiovascular diseases are the leading cause of death in individuals of both sexes in Brazil, accounting for 20% of all deaths in people over the age of 30 (MANSUR; FAVARATO, 2012), it is important to look for new therapeutic measures to prevent cardiovascular diseases. Among the most varied forms of treatment for these diseases, phytotherapy has really established itself as an effective and safe way, and green tea is an excellent herbal medicine with these properties.

Green tea is an important nutritional strategy in these cases because dyslipidemia is a determining factor in the development of cardiovascular diseases and one of the most studied forms of this tea today is its use, either naturally (folk medicine) or in capsules. Green tea has these properties due to the potent action of its polyphenols which limit lipid peroxidation, thus preventing the onset or controlling the rates for individuals with dyslipidemia.

From the analysis of all these studies that used green tea in humans or rodents, with various combinations, either with a normal diet for rodents or a cafeteria diet (high in fat), or in patients who had a fat-controlled diet or not, It can be concluded that this herbal medicine has significant effects in terms of lipid levels, with effects on lowering LDL, total cholesterol, increasing HDL, reducing weight and consequently BMI and thus improving health as a whole.

It can be concluded that green tea is one of the most effective natural ways to combat dyslipidemia, if combined with a balanced diet, and used regularly, thus reducing the chance of developing cardiovascular diseases in the future.

REFERENCES

BASU, A. et al. Green tea supplementation increases glutathione and plasma antioxidant capacity in adults with the metabolic syndrome. **Nutrition Research**, v. 33, p.180-187, 2013.

BATISTA, G. A. P. et al. Prospective double-blind crossover study of Camellia Sinensis (green tea) in dyslipidemias. **Arquivos Brasileiros de Cardiologia**, v. 93, n.2, p. 128-134, 2009.

BOSE, M. et al. The Major Green Tea Polyphenol, Epigallocatechin-3-Gallate, Inhibits Obesity, Metabolic Syndrome, and Fatty Liver Disease in High-Fat-Fed Mice. **Journal of Nutrition**, v.138, p.1677-1683, 2008.

HERNANDEZ-FIGUEROA, T.T.; RODRIGUEZ-RODRIGUEZ, E.; SANCHEZ- MUNIZ, F. J. The green tea, a good choice for cardiovascular disease prevention. **Archivos Latinoamericanos de Nutrición**, v. 54, n. 4, p. 380-94, 2004.

HOOPER, L. et al. Flavonoids, flavonoid-rich foods, and cardiovascular risk: a meta-analysis of randomized controlled trials. **American Journal of Clinical Nutrition**, v. 88, p. 38-50, 2008.

IBGE. Brazilian Institute of Geography and Statistics. Sociodemographic and Health Indicators in Brazil. **Studies and Research on Demographic and Socioeconomic Information**, n. 25, 2009.

KAO, Y.H.; HIIPAKKA, R. A.; LIAO, S. Modulation of Endocrine Systems and Food Intake by Green Tea Epigallocatechin Gallate. **Endocrinology**, v. 141, n. 3, p. 980-987, 2000.

MANSUR, P. A.; FAVARATO, D. Cardiovascular Disease Mortality in Brazil and in the Metropolitan Region of São Paulo. **Arquivos Brasileiros de Cardiologia**, v. 99, n. 2, p. 755-761, 2012.

MURASE, T. et al. Beneficial Effects of Tea Catechins on Diet-induced Obesity: Stimulation of Lipid Catabolism in the Liver. **International Journal of Obesity**, v. 26, n. 11, p. 1459-1464, 2002.

NAGAO, T. et al. Ingestion of a tea rich in catechins leads to a reduction in body fat and malondialdehyde-modified LDL in men. **American Journal of Clinical Nutrition**, v. 81, n. 1, p. 122-9, 2005.

NAGLE, D. G.; FERREIRA, D.; ZHOU, Y. Epigallocatechin-3-gallate (EGCG): chemical and biomedical perspectives. **Phytochemistry**, v. 67, n. 17, p. 1849-1855, 2006.

ONAKPOYA, I. et al. The effect of green tea on blood pressure and lipid profile: a systematic review and meta-analysis of randomized clinical trials. **Nutrition, Metabolism and Cardiovascular Diseases**, v.24, p. 823-836, 2014.

PARK, H. J. et al. Green tea extract attenuates hepatic steatosis by decreasing adipose lipogenesis and enhancing hepatic antioxidant defenses in ob/ob mice. **The Journal of Nutritional Biochemistry**, v. 22, p. 393-400, 2011.

PIMENTEL, C. V. M. B.; FRANCKI, V. M.; GOLLÜCKE, A. P. B. **Alimentos Funcionais:** Introdutão às principais substâncias bioativas em alimentos. Sao Paulo: Livraria Varela, p. 36-41, 2005.

RAEDERSTORFF, D. G. et al. Effect of EGCG on Lipid Absorption and Plasma Lipd Levels in Rats. **The Journal of Nutritional Biochemistry**, v. 14, n. 6, p. 326332, 2003.

SA, R. S.; TURELLA, T. K.; BETTEGA, J. M. P. R. **The effects of polyphenols: catechins and flavonoids from *Camellia sinensis* on skin ageing and lipid metabolism**. Course Conclusion Paper (Graduation in Cosmetology and Aesthetics) - Universidade do Vale do Itajai, Balneàrio Camboriù, 2007.

SCHMIDT, M. I. et al. Chronic non-communicable diseases in Brazil: current burden and challenges. **Saùde no Brasil**, v.4, p. 61-74, 2011.

SUZUKI-SUGIHARA, N. et al. Green tea catechins prevent low-density lipoprotein oxidation via their accumulation in low-density lipoprotein particles in humans. **Nutrition Research**, v.36, p.16-23, 2016.

TANG, J. et al. Tea consumption and mortality of all cancers, CVD and all causes: a meta-analysis of eighteen prospective cohort studies. **British Journal of Nutrition**, v.11, n. 4, p. 673-683, 2015.

TEIXEIRA, S. S.; ZANCANARO, V.; SANTOS, P. Efficacy of chronic use of green tea infusion (*Camellia sinensis*) in reducing total cholesterol, plasma LDL-cholesterol and body mass index in patients with hypercholesterolemia. **AGORA: Journal of Scientific Dissemination**, v. 16, n. 2, 2012.

YOKOZAWA, T.; NAKAGAWA, T.; KITANI, K. Antioxidative Activity of Green Tea Polyphenol in Cholesterol-Fed Rats. **Journal of Agricultural and Food Chemistry**, v. 50, n. 12, p. 3549-3552, 2002.

ZHENG, X. X. et al. Effects of green tea catechins with or without caffeine on glycemic control in adults: a meta-analysis of randomized controlled trials.

American Journal of Clinical Nutrition, v. 97, n. 129, p.750-762, 2013.

CHAPTER 10

CARDIOPROTECTIVE EFFECT OF GARLIC EXTRACT (*ALLIUM SATIVUM*): A REVIEW OF THE LITERATURE

Bruno Rafael Virginio de Sousa[1]

Hiarla Correia Wanderley[2]

Andreza Araùjo Duarte[3]

Yohanna de Oliveira[4]

1. Postgraduate student in Sports Nutrition, Faculdades Integradas de Patos (FIP);

2. Graduated in Nutrition, Mauricio de Nassau College, Campina Grande/PB;

3. Postgraduate student in Clinical and Functional Nutrition, Faculdades Integradas de Patos (FIP);

4. Master's student in Nutritional Sciences, Federal University of Paraiba.

ABSTRACT: Cardiovascular diseases (CVDs) are multifactorial pathologies considered to be one of the major causes of death in the world population. Among the new therapeutic alternatives that are being used to treat these diseases, the herb *Allium sativum*, popularly known as garlic, has demonstrated various cardioprotective effects in the coadjuvant treatment of pathologies related to CVDs. Its effects are attributed to its anti-hypertensive, anti-inflammatory and antioxidant activities. The aim of this study was to analyze the potential therapeutic effects of garlic (*Allium sativum*) on cardiovascular diseases. To this end, a bibliographical review was carried out focusing on studies that address the influence of garlic on cardiovascular diseases, using its extract. Based on research published in the Sciencedirect, PubMed and SciELO databases, only articles published in the last 8 years were considered. The results obtained showed that *Allium sativum* can indeed be considered a herbal medicine with cardioprotective properties. Therefore, it can be concluded that garlic has positive effects on various pathologies related to the cardiovascular system, and being low-cost, it facilitates access to the treatment of these diseases.

Keywords: Garlic extract. Cardiovascular disease. Herbal medicine.

1 INTRODUCTION

Cardiovascular diseases are classified as the main causes of death in the world's adult population and are also associated with various other comorbidities. According to the *American Heart Association*, the risk factors commonly associated with cardiovascular disease are dyslipidemia, obesity, hypertension, diabetes and smoking (CICHOCKI et al., 2017). In addition to these, the risk of cardiovascular events increases with age, as does the prevalence of metabolic syndrome (SOAR, 2015).

According to data from the World Health Organization (WHO), it has been noted that in recent decades, out of every 50 million deaths that are reported, 17 million, or 30% of them, are related to cardiovascular diseases (BUTLER, 2011).

Some aspects inherent to CVDs, such as the evolution of diagnostic methods, better pathophysiological knowledge of cardiac events, effective cardiovascular prevention measures and the use of new therapies, have made it possible to change the prognosis of CVDs. These tools contribute to increased survival and, consequently, to the emergence of possible comorbidities triggered by cardiovascular diseases (BRASIL, 2013; TARGHER; BYRNE, 2015). Among the new therapeutic alternatives that have emerged in recent years as an aid to more traditional treatments is the use of herbal medicines, which are defined as products derived from plants used for medicinal purposes and to promote health.

Among the herbal medicines that act on the cardiovascular system, one of the most prominent is garlic (*Allium sativum*), and in recent years the use of this plant species has increased substantially in order to help treat chronic non-communicable diseases (ALLISON; LOWE; RAHMAN, 2012). Its ability to reduce and/or prevent cardiovascular disease has been widely reported (ASDAQ; INAMDAR, 2010; SCHWINGSHACKL; MISSBACH; HOFFMANN, 2015; RAHMEN; LOWE; SMITH, 2016). This therapeutic capacity of garlic is attributed to sulfur-containing compounds, mainly allicin and S-allylcysteine, in addition, other organosulfur compounds, thiosulfinates, ajoenes present bioactive components responsible for improving the prognosis of various chronic diseases (SULERIA et al., 2015).

Therefore, the aim of this literature review was to analyze the potential therapeutic effects of garlic (*Allium sativum*) on cardiovascular diseases.

2 MATERIAL AND METHODS

This is a qualitative, descriptive, exploratory and cross-sectional study carried out using an integrative literature review, which involves searching for and analyzing several scientific articles on the chosen topic. For the bibliographic survey, searches were carried out in the electronic databases Sciencedirect, PubMed and SciELO. The keywords used to search for the articles were identified in the Health Sciences Descriptors (DECS), from which the following index terms were selected: "garlic extract", "Allium sativum", "cardiovascular diseases", "cardioprotective effects" and "phytotherapy".

By applying the index terms, 211 articles were obtained, of which 25 were selected to make up this review. The inclusion criteria were articles published in Portuguese, English or Spanish between 2009 and 2017, which dealt with cardiovascular diseases and the use of garlic extract (*Allium sativum*) as a therapeutic tool in the treatment of CVDs in adults and the elderly. As exclusion criteria, articles were discarded if they did not belong to the 2009 to 2017 timeframe, with scientific evidence in other pathologies. Figure (1) shows the flowchart of the article selection process.

Figure 1. Flowchart of the selection stages for the articles chosen for analysis.

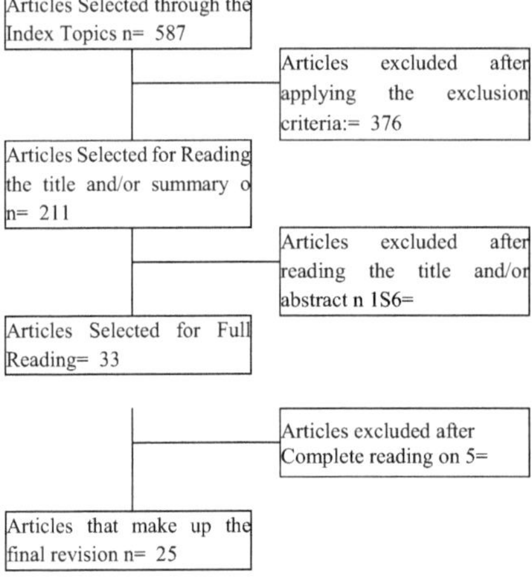

3 RESULTS AND DISCUSSION

3.1 Characteristics of cardiovascular diseases

The cardiovascular system can be classified as one of the most important systems in the body and is responsible for maintaining and regulating the survival of the human organism. It is made up of veins, arteries, arterioles, capillaries and the heart. Cardiac contractions are responsible for propelling the blood that is pumped throughout the body, carrying out the transportation of oxygen and nutrients that are necessary for the proper functioning of the cells (GUYTON; HALL, 2012).

The cardiovascular system is constantly exposed to numerous risk factors that can affect the body's homeostasis, causing unwanted changes in the biochemical, physiological and mechanical functions of the heart, thus causing cardiovascular diseases, and these risk factors can be both endogenous and exogenous (PITTHAN; MARTINS; BARBISAN, 2014).

Cardiovascular diseases are part of a group of acquired diseases that are interrelated with other series of pathologies in which CVD can develop, including: Coronary Artery Disease (CAD), Atherosclerosis, Systemic Arterial Hypertension (SAH), Ischemic Heart Disease, Vascular Disease Peripheral (PVD) and Heart Failure (HF) (MAHAN; ESCOTTSTUMP; RAYMOND, 2013).

There are two ways of preventing the disease: primary prevention, which involves addressing and resolving the risk factors that may or may not exist in people with CVD, such as sedentary lifestyles, blood pressure levels and total cholesterol and its fractions, among others. And secondary prevention, which deals with both nutritional and pharmacological care to prevent the worsening of the disease and the inflammatory process (KUEHLEIN et al., 2010). Nutritional care includes phytotherapy as an important therapeutic measure, used more frequently nowadays (EKOR, 2014).

3.2 Cardioprotective properties of garlic (*Allium sativum*)

Garlic exerts its therapeutic effects due to the presence of more than 200 chemical compounds. This plant contains sulphur compounds (allicin, alliin and ajoenes), volatile oils, enzymes (allinase, peroxidase and miracinase), carbohydrates (sucrose and glucose), minerals (selenium), amino acids such as cisterna, glutamine, isoleucine and methionine which help protect cells from free radical damage (KHATUA; ADELA; BANERJEE, 2013).

Its composition contains large quantities of organosulfur compounds, which act as cardioprotectants, modulating the expression of adhesion molecules, as well as the enzyme endothelial nitric oxide synthase, among other mechanisms (BARBOSA; FERNANDES, 2014). Table (1) shows some recent studies on the cardioprotective effects of garlic.

Table 1. Studies on the effect of garlic on the cardiovascular system.

Authors	Type of study	Methods	Results
Mahdavi-Roshan et al. (2015)	Randomized, double-blind, placebo-controlled.	70 patients aged 25 to 75 with severe coronary artery disease undergoing angioplasty. Administration of 1200 mg of allicin twice a day, in tablets,	After three months of treatment, there was a reduction in the thickness of the carotid intima-media layer in the treated group, to the detriment of the

		started three days after angioplasty.	increase observed in the placebo group.
Jung et al. (2014)	Randomized, double blind, placebo-controlled.	55 volunteers with hypercholesterolemia. Administration of 3 g of black garlic extract twice a day before a morning meal for 12 weeks.	There was no significant difference in triglyceride, total cholesterol and LDL levels between the groups. However, ApoB, HDL and LDL/ApoB increased in the supplemented group.
Orekhov et al. (2013)	Randomized, double-blind, placebo-controlled.	196 men aged between 40 and 74, with the onset of atherosclerosis in the carotid artery and who were not taking medication. Administration of 150 mg of garlic extract or placebo, 2 times a day.	Garlic treatment had a beneficial impact on early atherosclerosis in the carotid arteries. In the placebo group, however, the progression of atherosclerosis prevailed.
Ried; Frank; Stocks (2013)	Randomized, double-blind, placebo-controlled.	79 participants with uncontrolled systemic hypertension, for 12 weeks. Administration of 480mg of aged garlic extract +1.2mg of S-allicysteine twice a day.	The dose applied significantly reduced systemic blood pressure compared to placebo. The reduction is comparable to that achieved by antihypertensive drugs.
Ahmadi et al. (2013)	Randomized, double-blind, placebo-controlled.	60 patients, aged 40 to 79, who received chronic statin therapy. Administration of 250 mg of aged garlic once a day for one year.	Risks of progression of coronary artery calcification, changes in epicardial white and brown adipose tissue and increased homocysteine were significantly lower in the garlic-supplemented group than in the placebo group ($p<0.05$).
Lau et al. (2013)	Clinical, Randomized.	125 patients were recruited with a history of ischemic stroke due to an atherothrombotic process. Half were given a diet containing more than 3.37g/day of garlic, and the other half were given a diet low in garlic.	The study showed that among patients with ischemic stroke, daily intake of garlic had a significant positive correlation with endothelial function. A decrease in blood triglyceride levels was also noted.
Sobenin et al. (2010)	Randomized, double-blind,	51 patients with coronary disease over 12 months.	Garlic treatment caused an increase in triglycerides,
	placebo-controlled.	Administer 150 mg of garlic tablets twice a day.	although it did lower cholesterol and LDL. It was concluded that the 10-year prognostic risk of myocardial infarction decreased considerably.
Ried; Frank; Stocks (2010)	Randomized, double-blind, placebo-	50 with uncontrolled hypertension. Daily administration for 12 weeks of	Aged garlic extract is superior to placebo in reducing SBP in a similar

	controlled.	960 mg of garlic extract containing 2.4 mg of S-allylcysteine in the Treatment Group (GT) and placebo in the Control Group (GC).	way to current first-line drugs in patients with treated but uncontrolled hypertension.
Sobenin et al. (2009)	Randomized, double-blind, placebo-controlled.	84 newly diagnosed patients with mild to moderate hypertension. The garlic group was given 300 mg of garlic extract twice a day and the other group was given placebo for 8 weeks.	Garlic extract produced a statistically significant hypotensive effect on systemic and diastolic blood pressure in men with mild to moderate hypertension.

3.3 Effect of garlic on diseases interrelated with cardiovascular disease

3.3.1 Atherosclerosis

Atherosclerotic heart disease involves the loss of elasticity and narrowing of the blood vessel wall, caused by the accumulation of fatty plaques. These fatty plaques are commonly formed during the inflammation process, which is stimulated by the phagocytic response of monocytes (white blood cells). The monocytes in the tissues develop into macrophages, which ingest the cholesterol that has been oxidized and turn into cells called foam cells and, subsequently, into fatty streaks in these vessels (MAHAN; ESCOTT-STUMP; RAYMOND, 2013).

Regarding this disease, aged garlic extract with micronutrient supplementation (EAE-S) is associated with a lack of progression of coronary atherosclerosis, as well as improving vascular function and showing beneficial effects on oxidative stress biomarkers (BUDOFF et al., 2009; AHMADI et al., 2013). A randomized study carried out over 12 months with 60 asymptomatic individuals aged between 40 and 79 who had a Framingham Risk (FR) of 10-20% and Coronary Artery Calcification (CAC) > 30 who received chronic statin treatment without clinical coronary artery disease (CAD), found that the group supplemented with 250 mg of aged garlic extract and micronutrients had significantly lower risks of CAD progression, changes in epicardial white and brown adipose tissue and an increase in homocysteine compared to the placebo group ($p<0.05$) (AHMADI et al., 2013). Improving these variables attenuates the progression of atherosclerotic plaque, improving the prognosis of CAD.

Another recent randomized, placebo-controlled clinical study was carried out on 56 patients with CAD aged between 25 and 75 years. The patients were divided into two groups: the garlic group (n=27), receiving garlic powder tablets (1200 mg of allicin) twice a day, and the placebo group (n=29), receiving cornstarch tablets for 3 months. As a result, after 3 months of intervention, the values of the Carotid Intima Media Thickness (CIMT) showed smaller variations (0.009± 0.007 mm). In the placebo group, there was an increase in CIMT values (0.04± 0.01 mm) compared to the beginning of the study. After 3 months of treatment, the mean EIMC difference was significant between the two groups ($p<0.001$). However, no relevant differences were observed in the concentration of plasma lipids and lipoproteins (total cholesterol, triglycerides, LDL, HDL, Apolipoprotein Al and Apolipoprotein B) between the two groups (MAHDAVI-ROSHAN et al., 2015).

Koyoshi et al. (2011) reinforce these results, as their study found that patients with CAD had a significantly thicker IMT than the non-CAD group.

In fact, garlic, like other herbal medicines when used properly, has anti-inflammatory functions with the ability to inhibit and/or prevent the onset and progression of atherosclerosis, and its anti-inflammatory capacity is attributed to the concentrations of organosulphur compounds which are extremely important for protecting the walls of blood vessels, making it a food of great importance in the prevention of cardiovascular diseases (TSAI et al., 2012).

3.3.2 Hypertension

Hypertension is characterized by persistently high blood pressure levels. This level is considered high when Systolic Blood Pressure (SBP) is greater than or equal to 140 mmHg and Diastolic Blood Pressure (DBP) is greater than or equal to 90 mmHg. This elevation is often associated with functional and metabolic changes in the heart, brain, kidneys and blood vessels (BRASIL, 2010). Studies have shown positive effects of garlic extract on blood pressure values, thus helping to treat hypertension (NAKASONE et al., 2012; RIED; FRANK; STOCKS, 2013; ASDAQ; INAMDAR, 2010; SCHWINGSHACKL; MISSBACH; HOFFMANN, 2015).

A meta-analysis carried out by Ried (2016) analyzed 20 trials with a total of 970 participants. Overall, the individuals showed an average decrease in SBP of 5.1 ± 2.2 mmHg ($p<0.001$) and an average decrease in DBP of 2.5 ± 1.6 mmHg ($p<0.002$) compared to placebo. When analyzing the subgroups of hypertensive patients, at the start of the study there was a more significant reduction in SBP of 8.7 ± 2.2 mmHg ($p<0.001$) in 10 studies, to the detriment of a reduction in DBP of 6.1 ± 1.3 mmHg ($p<0.001$) in 6 studies. This meta-analysis also showed that the trials demonstrated an effect of garlic on lowering total cholesterol and on the immune system.

Shouk et al. (2014) reinforced these results from their review which found antihypertensive effects of garlic and its derivatives. The study analyzed the bioactive compounds in garlic and the various parameters involved in the pathogenesis of hypertension. It became clear that recent scientific advances are centered on alpha-allyl-cysteine and allicin as modulators of various parameters implicated in hypertension. These parameters include oxidative stress, oxide bioavailability, hydrogen sulphide production, angiotensin-converting enzyme activity and expression of the nuclear transcription factor Kappa Beta.

3.3.3 Dyslipidemia

Dyslipidemia is characterized by changes in lipid levels and, according to the 2013 Brazilian Dyslipidemia Guidelines, it can be classified into 4 types: isolated hypercholesterolemia, where there is only an increase in LDL-C; elevated hypertriglyceridemia, increased TG values; mixed hyperlipidemia, in which both LDL-C and TG values are elevated; and low HDL-C, where there is a decrease in HDL-C alone or associated with an increase in TG and/or LDL-C levels (BRASIL, 2013).

In a randomized, double-blind, placebo-controlled clinical trial that aimed to assess whether a dietary supplement containing fermented garlic decreased serum lipid concentrations in volunteers with mild hyperlipidemia, 55 apparently healthy individuals with serum triglyceride concentrations between 120 and 200 mg/dL were randomly divided into two groups, one ingesting Fermented Garlic (FA) and the other ingesting placebo capsules, for 12 weeks. During the intervention period, it was observed that the intake of FA significantly reduced triglyceride levels ($p=0.062$), total cholesterol ($p=0.003$), LDL cholesterol levels ($p=0.001$) and the LDL/HDL ratio ($p<0.001$) (HIGASHIKAWA et al., 2012).

Jung et al. (2014) found in their study with 55 participants divided into two groups: Garlic ($n=28$) and placebo ($n=27$), that black garlic extract ingested twice a day (total 6 g/day) before the consumption of a meal every morning for 12 weeks, did not imply significant differences in the concentrations of triglycerides, LDL, total cholesterol or free fatty acids (FFA) between the two groups. However, garlic extract did increase HDL levels compared to the placebo group at the end of the study. In addition, a significant decrease in apoprotein B levels and an increase in the LDL-C/apoB ratio were observed in the garlic group. It was concluded that garlic extract supplementation at this dose has a cardioprotective effect by reducing atherogenic markers in patients with hypercholesterolemia.

3.3.4 Garlic and other diseases with cardiovascular associations

In addition to all the diseases already mentioned, garlic extract has a proven effect on a number of other pathologies involved directly or indirectly with the cardiovascular system.

In the case of heart failure (HF), garlic has been shown to be beneficial in treating the condition, as it is able to normalize hemodynamic parameters, improving systolic and diastolic blood pressure and generating better blood flow (SANTIAGO et al., 2009).

In a study carried out with rats, in which norepinephrine (NE) was injected to induce cardiomyocyte hypertrophy, followed by garlic extract in order to analyze the reduction in the death of these cells caused by NE, garlic showed a significant reduction in the increase in size and death of cardiomyocytes, as well as a reduction in the oxidative stress that was also caused in cardiac muscle cells when NE was applied (LOUIS et al., 2012).

It has also been shown in an animal model (n=10) that pretreatment with extract of fermented garlic can be useful as an efficient therapeutic strategy for preventing ischemic/reperfusion myocardial injury in H9c2 cells (LEE et al., 2017).

On the other hand, Rahman, Lowe and Smith (2016) investigated the effects of Aged Garlic Extract (EAE) on intra-platelet cell signaling and platelet shape change with 14 volunteers in their study. Platelet aggregation was induced by Adenosine Diphosphate (ADP) in the presence of EAE up to a concentration of 6.25% (vol:vol) alone or in combination with 3-morpholinosidnonimine (Sin-1). As a result, garlic extract decreased platelet aggregation at all concentrations tested, this decrease was more pronounced in the presence of Sin-1 and ranged from 15% to 67%. These results indicate that EAE inhibits platelet aggregation by increasing cyclic nucleotides and inhibiting fibrinogen binding, in addition to altering platelet shape.

Butt et al. (2009) demonstrated in their studies with dyslipidemic individuals that garlic has antioxidant activity, because the nutritional components present in it are able to protect cells against the effects of free radicals, having the ability to eliminate these radicals and protect the membrane from damage while maintaining its cellular integrity. With this antioxidant activity, garlic is able to inactivate reactive oxygen species, increasing the activity of cellular antioxidant enzymes (SANTIAGO et al., 2009).

In addition to the various studies with positive results from garlic extract, Vazquez-Pietro et al. (2011) were able to demonstrate that the organosulfur compounds present in garlic act to modulate the expression of adhesion molecules, as well as enzymes such as the enzyme endothelial nitric oxide synthase. In their study, 30 male rats were given oral doses of 150 mg/kg/day and 400 mg/kg/day respectively of aqueous extracts of garlic and onion over a period of 14 weeks. It was observed that supplementation with garlic and onion extracts reduced oxidative stress and increased the activity of the enzyme nitric oxide synthase, as well as attenuating the expression of VCAM-1. By reducing oxidative stress, garlic has also been shown to be effective in reducing the infarcted area (SANTIAGO et al., 2009).

In general, the literature shows positive effects of garlic on diseases and comorbidities associated with the cardiovascular system. This is important because, through phytotherapy, new alternatives for the treatment of cardiovascular diseases are frequently appearing and garlic is one of these herbal medicines whose benefits have been proven without any major undesirable effects.

4 CONCLUSIONS

Cardiovascular diseases are in fact the world's greatest concern in terms of Chronic Non-Communicable Diseases (CNCD), a problem which has led science to incessantly search for alternatives to minimize the burden caused by CVDs. The use of plants with proven phytotherapeutic properties is an alternative means of treating these diseases, especially garlic (*Allium sativum*), which contains bioactive compounds with cardioprotective properties.

This review shows that garlic has positive effects on blood pressure, blood lipid fractions, anti-platelet and antioxidant activity, as well as improving atherosclerosis, acute myocardial infarction, heart failure and coronary artery disease. Therefore, garlic is an excellent low-cost herbal medicine for treating CVD that can be used safely, but under the prescription of a specialized professional.

REFERENCES

AHMADI, N. et al. Aged garlic extract with supplement is associated with increase in brown adipose, decrease in white adipose tissue and predict lack of progression in coronary atherosclerosis. **International Journal of Cardiology**, v. 168, n. 3, p. 2310-2314, 2013.

ALLISON, G. L.; LOWE, M. G.; RAHMAN, K. Aged garlic extract inhibits platelet activation by increasing intracellular cAMP and reducing the interaction of GPIIb/IIIa receptor with fibrinogen. **Life Science**, v. 91, p. 1275-80, 2012.

ASDAQ, S. M.; INAMDAR, M. N. Potential of garlic and its active constituent, S- allyl cysteine, as antihypertensive and cardioprotective in presence of captopril. **Phytomedicine**, v. 17, n. 13, p. 1016-1026, 2010.

BARBOSA, T. N. R.; FERNANDES, D. C. Bioactive compounds and cardiovascular diseases: reviewing the scientific evidence. **Estudos**, v. 41, n. 2, p. 181192, 2014.

BRAZIL. Brazilian Society of Cardiology. V Brazilian Guideline on Dyslipidemias and Prevention of Atherosclerosis. **Arquivos Brasileiros de Cardiologia**, v. 101, n. 4, 2013.

BRAZIL. Brazilian Society of Hypertension. VI Brazilian Hypertension Guidelines. **Revista Hipertensâo**, v. 13, n. 1, 2010.

BUDOFF, M. J. et al. Aged garlic extract supplemented with B vitamins, folic acid and L-arginine retards the progression of subclinical atherosclerosis: a randomized clinical trial. **Preventive Medicine**, v. 49, n. 2, p. 101-107, 2009.

BUTLER, D. International summit considers how to stem the rise in noncommunicable diseases. **Nature**, v. 447, p. 260-261, 2015.

BUTT, M. S. et al. Garlic: nature's protection against physiological threats.

Critical Reviews in Food Science and Nutrition, v. 49, n. 6, p. 538-551, 2009.

CICHOCKI, M. et al. Physical activity and modulation of cardiovascular risk. **Brazilian Journal of Sports Medicine**, v. 23, n. 1, p. 21-25, 2017.

EKOR, M. The growing use of herbal medicines: issues relating to adverse reactions and challenges in monitoring safety. **Frontiers in Pharmacology**, v. 4, p. 177, 2014.

GUYTON, A. C.; HALL, J. E. **Fundamentals of Physiology**. Rio de Janeiro, Elsevier, 2012.

HIGASHIKAWA, F. et al. Reduction of serum lipids by the intake of the extract of garlic fermented with Monascus pilosus: a randomized, double-blind, placebo- controlled clinical trial. **Clinical Nutrition**, v. 31, n. 2, p. 261-266, 2012.

JUNG, E. S. et al. Reduction of blood lipid parameters by a 12-week supplementation of aged black garlic: A randomized controlled trial. **Nutrition**, v. 30, n. 9, p. 1034-1039, 2014.

KHATUA, T. N.; ADELA, R.; BANERJEE, S. K. Garlic and cardioprotection: insights into the molecular mechanisms. **Canadian Journal of Physiology and Pharmacology**, v. 91, n. 6, p. 448-458, 2013.

KOYOSHI, R. et al. Clinical significance of flow-mediated dilation, brachial intima-media thickness and pulse wave velocity in patients with and without coronary artery disease. **Circulation Journal**, v. 76, n. 6, p. 1469-1475, 2011.

KUEHLEIN, T. et al. Quaternary prevention: a task of the general practitioner. **Primary Care**, v.10, n. 18, p 350-354, 2010.

LAU, K. K. et al. Garlic intake is an independent predictor of endothelial function in patients with ischemic stroke. **The Journal of Nutrition, Health & Aging**, v. 17, n. 7, p. 600-604, 2013.

LEE, Y. J. et al. Potential protective effects of fermented garlic extract on myocardial ischemia-reperfusion injury utilizing in vitro and ex vivo models. **Journal of Functional Foods**, v. 33, p. 278-285, 2017.

LOUIS, X. L. et al. Garlic extracts prevent oxidative stress, hypertrophy and apoptosis in cardiomyocytes: a role for nitric oxide and hydrogen sulfide. **BMC**

Complementary and Alternative Medicine, v. 12, n.140, 2012.

MAHAN, L. K.; ESCOTT-STUMP, S.; RAYMOND, J. L. **Krause: Food, Nutrition and Diet Therapy**. 13ª ed. Rio de Janeiro: Elsevier, 2013.

MAHDAVI-ROSHAN, M. et al. Effect of garlic powder tablet on carotid intimamedia thickness in patients with coronary artery disease. **Nutrition and Health**, v. 22, n. 2, p. 143-155, 2015.

NAKASONE, Y. et al. Effect of a traditional Japanese garlic preparation on blood pressure in prehypertensive and mildly hypertensive adults. **Experimental and Therapeutic Medicine**, v. 5, n. 2, p. 399-405, 2012.

OREKHOV, A. N. et al. Anti-atherosclerotic therapy based on botanicals. **Recent Patents on Cardiovascular Drug Discovery**, v. 8, n. 1, p. 56, 2013.

PITTHAN, E.; MARTINS, O. M. O.; BARBISAN, J. N. New inflammatory and endothelial dysfunction biomarkers: cardiovascular risk prediction. **Revista da AMRIGS**, v. 58, n. 1, p. 69-77, 2014.

RAHMAN, K.; LOWE, G. M.; SMITH, S. Aged Garlic Extract Inhibits Human Platelet Aggregation by Altering Intracellular Signaling and Platelet Shape Change. **The Journal of Nutrition**, v. 146, p. 410-415, 2016.

RIED, K. Garlic Lowers Blood Pressure in Hypertensive Individuals, Regulates Serum Cholesterol, and Stimulates Immunity: An Updated Meta-analysis and Review. **Journal of Nutrition**, v. 146, n. 2, p. 389-396, 2016.

RIED, K.; FRANK, O. R.; STOCKS, N. P. Aged garlic extract reduces blood pressure in hypertensives: a dose-response trial. **European Journal of Clinical Nutrition**, v. 67, n. 1, p. 64-70, 2013.

RIED, K.; FRANK, O. R.; STOCKS, N. P. Aged garlic extract lowers blood pressure in patients with treated but uncontrolled hypertension: a randomized controlled trial. **Maturitas**, v. 67, n. 2, p. 144-150, 2010.

SANTIAGO, M. B. et al. Effect of Allium sativum administration on cardiovascular alterations in Wistar rats with myocardial infarction. **Revista de Ciências Farmacêuticas Bàsica e Aplicada**, v. 30, n. 1, p. 75-82, 2009.

SCHWINGSHACKL, L.; MISSBACH, B.; HOFFMANN, G. An umbrella review of garlic intake and risk of cardiovascular disease. **Phytomedicine**, v. 23, n. 11, p. 1127-1133, 2015.

SHOUK, R. et al. Mechanisms underlying the antihypertensive effects of garlic bioactives. **Nutrition Research**, v. 34, n. 2, p. 106-115, 2014.

SOAR, C. Prevalence of cardiovascular risk factors in non-institutionalized elderly. **Revista Brasileira de Geriatria e Gerontologia**, v. 18, n. 2, p. 385-395, 2015.

SOBENIN, I. A. et al. The effects of time-released garlic powder tablets on multifunctional cardiovascular risk in patients with coronary artery disease. **Lipids in Health and Disease**, v. 9, n. 1, p. 1, 2010.

SOBENIN, I. A. et al. Time-released garlic powder tablets lower systolic and diastolic blood pressure in men with mild and moderate arterial hypertension.

Hypertension Research, v. 32, n. 6, p. 433-437, 2009.

SULERIA, H. A. R. et al. Garlic (Allium sativum): diet based therapy of 21st century-a review. **Asian Pacific Journal Of Tropical Disease**, v. 5, n. 4, p. 271278, 2015.

TARGHER, G.; BYRNE, C. D. Circulating markers of liver function and cardiovascular disease risk. **Arteriosclerosis, Thrombosis, and Vascular Biology**, v. 35, n. 11, p. 2290-2296, 2015.

TSAI, C. W. et al. Garlic: Health benefits and actions. **BioMedicine**, v. 2, n. 1, p. 17-29, 2012.

VAZQUEZ-PRIETO, M.A. et al. Garlic and Onion Attenuates Vascular Inflammation and Oxidative Stress in Fructose-Fed Rats. **Journal of Nutrition and Metabolism**, p. 1-7, 2011.

CHAPTER 11

CHAMOMILE (*MATRICARIA RECUTITA* L.) AND ITS THERAPEUTIC PROPERTIES: A REVIEW

Cristiane Félix Alves[1]

Maria das Graças Silva[2]

1. Nursing undergraduate student at Santa Emilia de Rodat College;

2. Master's Degree in Natural and Synthetic Bioactive Products, Federal University of Paraiba.

SUMMARY: Chamomile is a medicinal plant of European origin, with digestive and calming properties. Industrially, chamomile is used to extract its essence, which is widely used as a flavoring in the composition of soaps, perfumes and lotions, while chamomile extract and essence are used in the preparation of a wide variety of foods and beverages, and it is considered to be the most cultivated medicinal plant in the world. Therefore, the aim of this study was to gather data on chamomile, its characteristics, therapeutic properties and ways of using it. It was an exploratory bibliographical review with qualitative objectives. Camazulene, present in the plant's essential oil, has recognized anti-inflammatory activity, reinforced by the presence of matricin and α-bisabolol, with α-bisabolol having antiphlogistic, antibacterial, antimycotic and mucosal protective properties, thus acting against ulcers. We can conclude that chamomile is used for dyspepsia, flatulence and nausea, especially when gastrointestinal disorders are associated with nervous disorders. It is also used for nasal mucus and restlessness. Widely used in babies and children as a mild sedative, and for the treatment of colic and teething pain. It has been used topically for hemorrhoids, mastitis and leg ulcers. It has essential oils and flavonoids and is used in folk medicine for its anti-inflammatory, carminative and spasmolytic properties. The anti-inflammatory and antispasmodic actions are related to the main properties found in the essential oil, namely the sesquiterpenes, which are derivatives of bisabolol and guaianolid lactones (procamazulene), and the spasmolytic property to the flavonoids. The plant's chemical constituents, around 120, have been identified in chamomile as secondary metabolites, including 28 terpenoids, 36 flavonoids and 52 additional compounds with potent pharmacological activity.

Keywords: Chamomile. Therapeutic properties. Digestive. Soothing.

1 INTRODUCTION

Nowadays, there has been a reformulation of the lifestyle of society as a whole, in which natural and ecological values are being revived, with great intensity, in the specification of new concepts in all sectors of practical daily life and scientific knowledge. In this way, the use of plants for medicinal purposes has restored and aroused interest in the knowledge of the main characteristics of the medicines produced, including their chemical composition, morphology, pharmacological properties, among others (ARGENTA et al., 2011).

Plants are used as the only therapeutic resource by a portion of the Brazilian population and more than two thirds of the world's population. The main factors influencing the maintenance of this practice are the low cost of plants and the high cost of medicines (ARGENTA et al., 2011).

However, for plants to be used properly for medicinal purposes, they need to meet all the criteria for quality, safety and efficacy, as well as having reproducible therapeutic properties and consistency in their chemical composition (OLIVEIRA, 2012).

Chamomile (*Chamomilla recutita* L.), synonym (*Matricaria chamomilla* L.) belongs to the Asteraceae family and is also known as perennial chamomile or Roman chamomile (ITF, 2008).

Chamomile is a very popular plant in Brazil, even though it is cultivated to a greater extent in North America. Among other uses, the plant is used for healing, perfume and food. Its most common form of use is tea, which is an infusion with digestive and calming properties (OLIVEIRA, 2012).

Chamomile is a herbaceous, annual and aromatic plant, native to the countryside of Western Asia and Southern Europe and is easily found in countries with a temperate climate. It has an erect stem, narrow leaves that are widely divided into thin, numerous segments. Tiny yellow flowers cluster together to form a central inflorescence. The central flowers are hermaphrodite, with a yellow, tubular corolla, and the marginal flowers are female with a white, ligulate corolla.

(ONOFRE; HARTMANN, 2010).

It is one of the oldest plants used in traditional European medicine and is now included in the Pharmacopoeias of almost all countries. Its emmenagogue action was discovered empirically by Dioscorides in ancient Greece and scientifically proven 2,000 years later (LORENZI;

MATOS, 2008).

The justification for this study was to deepen our knowledge of chamomile, its characteristics and phytotherapeutic properties, which are of great interest to the pharmaceutical, cosmetics and food industries.

Therefore, the main focus of this study was to analyse the following question: What does the specialized literature say about the medicinal properties of chamomile and how is it characterized phytotherapeutically? As a study hypothesis, we can state that chamomile is a plant widely used in the medicinal and cosmetic fields. Its therapeutic and pharmacological properties are based on its anti-inflammatory and astringent action. It acts as an antiseptic, anti-inflammatory, antioxidant, healing, refreshing, soothing, spot lightening, dermopurifying, brightening and improves skin capillarity.

Therefore, the general objective of this study was to gather data on chamomile, its characteristics, therapeutic properties and ways of using it. The specific objectives were to learn about and characterize chamomile as a medicinal plant, to identify how this herb is used, its main characteristics and medicinal properties, and to reflect on the use of chamomile in the treatment of certain illnesses.

2 MATERIAL AND METHODS

This study is an exploratory bibliographical review of a qualitative nature. Regarding bibliographical research, Kant (2007) states that, "it is present in all academic work, since it is at this stage of the work that the theme or phenomenon under discussion is theoretically founded".

Thus, it can be said that this bibliographical study used *already* published material, consisting of books and national articles, totaling 20 articles selected to make up this review, of which the inclusion criteria were all those related to the topic and the exclusion criteria were articles that were not intended to meet the research objectives. The descriptors used in the selection were: chamomile, therapeutic properties, digestive and calming.

3 RESULTS AND DISCUSSION

Chamomile is a plant that can adapt to almost any type of terrain. It is an annual herbaceous grass that grows to an average height of 30 to 50 cm. It has small flowers that look like little white daisies with a yellow core, which exude a delicate aroma and adorn pots and flowerbeds. Its stem is branched and its leaves are very jagged, similar to those of daisies, so that in the center is the inflorescence in chapters, orange-yellow in color, conical and hollow surrounded by white bracts (CORTEZ et al., 2007).

Of European origin, chamomile grows well in mild climates, but is capable of adapting to other environments, as long as the climate is not too hot. As well as being an ornamental plant, it produces a digestive and calming tea, soothing the skin and beautifying the hair (OLIVEIRA, 2012).

Industrially, chamomile is used to extract its essence, which is widely used as a flavoring in the composition of soaps, perfumes and lotions, while chamomile extract and essence are used in the preparation of a wide variety of foods and beverages and is considered to be the most cultivated medicinal plant in the world (LORENZI; MATOS, 2008).

The flowering tops of this plant contain essential oils and flavonoids and are used in folk medicine for their anti-inflammatory, carminative and spasmolytic properties. The anti-inflammatory and antispasmodic actions are related to the main properties found in the essential oil, namely the sesquiterpenes, which are derivatives of bisabolol and guaianolid Iactones (procamazulene), and the spasmolytic property to the flavonoids (OLIVEIRA, 2012).

The main chemical constituents of chamomile are: Blue essential oil - camazulene and camaviolin, α-bisabolol, immunostimulant polysaccharides, bicyclic ethers with spasmolytic action, flavonoids with bacteriostatic and trichomicidal action (luteolin, quercetin and rutin), and apigenin with anxiolytic and sedative action (FALKOWSKI; JACOMASSI; TAKEMURA, 2009).

Chamomile is used in both scientific and folk medicine, in the form of infusions and decoctions, as a bitter tonic, digestive aid, sedative, to facilitate the elimination of gas, combat colic and stimulate appetite. It also acts topically by applying warm compresses of the infusion to the abdomen to treat colic in children (LORENZI; MATOS, 2008).

Chamomile is also used for dyspepsia, flatulence and nausea, especially when gastrointestinal disorders are associated with nervous disorders. It is also used for nasal mucus and restlessness. Chamomile is widely used in babies and children as a mild sedative, and for the treatment of colic and teething pain. It has been used topically for hemorrhoids, mastitis and leg ulcers (DUARTE; LIMA, 2003).

The aqueous infusion of the flowers or the essential oil itself are also used in ointments and creams, and in pharmaceutical preparations for external use used to promote healing of the skin, relieve inflammation of the gums and as an antiviral in the treatment of herpes, properties which are mainly due to α-bisabolol (LORENZI; MATOS, 2008).

The plant's chemical constituents, especially the essential oil, are mainly located in the secretory channels and individual multicellular glands situated in the flower and receptacle. Around 120 chemical constituents have been identified in chamomile as secondary metabolites, including 28 terpenoids, 36 flavonoids and 52 additional compounds with potent pharmacological activity (ONOFRE; HARTMANN, 2010).

The popular use of chamomile in conventional medicine is so widespread that in Germany it was declared the most important medicinal plant in 1987. Its pharmacological effect is mainly related to its essential oil. Throughout its history, chamomile has been used to treat inflammatory disorders, menstrual pain, fever, diarrhea, intestinal tumors, soothing and also as an active ingredient used in ointments for atopic dermatitis (DUARTE; LIMA, 2003).

Pharmacological research into many components of the essential oil of German chamomile has shown positive results, such as bisabolol, which reduces inflammation and arthritis, prevents the development of gastric ulcers and acts against fungi and bacteria. Other examples are camazulene and matricin sesquiterpenes, for their anti-inflammatory action. In the case of camazulene, this effect can be understood by its inhibitory action on the concentration of neutrophilic granulocytes and leukotriene, as well as its antioxidant properties. In this sense, Sazegar et al. (2010 apud WILLIAMSON; DRIVER; BAXTER, 2012) analyzed the anti-oxidant effect of chamomile essential oil, observing its action in reactions involving free radicals.

Awang (1999 apud WILLIAMSON; DRIVER; BAXTER, 2012) states that the anti-inflammatory principle of chamomile components, in decreasing order of effectiveness, begins with apigenin, followed by matricin, camazulene and α-bisabolol. The author also points out that, in the technique used to obtain chamomile tea, only a small portion of the volatile oil, approximately 10%, and around 30% of the flavonoids are removed in this way.

In the study carried out by Alireza (2011 apud WILLIAMSON; DRIVER; BAXTER, 2012), he explains that the antimicrobial activity of the volatile oil was obtained with an inhibitory effect of close to 100% on gram-positive bacteria and 80% on gram-negative bacteria.

4 CONCLUSIONS

Finally, it should be noted that Europeans use chamomile in a wide variety of products, generally consumed as a tea herb and sold in the form of sachets or inflorescences. Information indicates that more than a million cups of chamomile tea are consumed every day throughout Europe.

It was therefore concluded that chamomile is used for dyspepsia, flatulence and nausea, especially when gastrointestinal disorders are associated with nervous disorders. It is also used for nasal mucus and restlessness. Widely used in babies and children as a mild sedative, and for the treatment of colic and teething pain. It has been used topically for hemorrhoids, mastitis and leg ulcers. It has essential oils and flavonoids and is used in folk medicine for its anti-inflammatory, carminative and spasmolytic properties. The anti-inflammatory and antispasmodic actions are related to the main properties found in the essential oil, namely the sesquiterpenes, which are derivatives of bisabolol and guaianolid lactones (procamazulene), and the spasmolytic property to the flavonoids.

REFERENCES

ARGENTA, S. C. et al. Medicinal plants: popular culture versus science. **Revista Vivências**, v. 7, n. 12, p. 51-60, 2011.

CORTEZ, L. E. R. et al. Quality control of chamomile sold in Maringà - Paranâ. **Proceedings of the V EPCC Encontro Internacional de Produçâo Cientifica Cesumar**, Maringà - PR, 2007.

DUARTE, M. R.; LIMA, M. P. Anâlise Farmacopéica de Amostras de Camomila - Matricaria recutita L., Asteraceae. **Visâo Acadêmica**, v. 4, n. 2, p. 89-92, 2003.

FALKOWSKI, G. J. S.; JACOMASSI, E.; TAKEMURA, O. S. Quality and authenticity of chamomile tea samples (Matricaria recutita L. - Asteraceae). **Revista do Instituto Adolfo Lutz**, v. 68, n. 1, p. 64-72, 2009.

ITF. ìndice **TERAPÈUTICO FITOTERAPICO**. ιª ed., Petrópolis, Rio de Janeiro: Editora EPUB, 2008. 328p.

KANT, I. **Metodologia do traballio cientifico**. 23ª ed. Sao Paulo: Artmed, 2007.

LORENZI, H.; MATOS, F. J. A. **Plantas medicinais no Brasil nativas e exóticas**. 2a ed. Nova Odessa-SP: Instituto Plantarum, 2008.

OLIVEIRA, B. P. **Content and chemical composition of essential oil in commercial samples of chamomile (*Matricaria chamomilla* L.)**. Dissertation (Master's Degree in Agrochemistry) - Federal University of Viçosa, Viçosa-Minas Gerais, 2012.

ONOFRE, S. B.; HARTMANN, K. C. Antimicrobial activity of chamomile essential oils (*Matricaria chamomilla* L.). **Revista Saùde e Pesquisa**, v. 3, n. 3, p. 279-284, 2010.

WILLIAMSON, E.; DRIVER, S.; BAXTER, K. **Stockley's drug interactions: medicinal plants and herbal medicines**. Porto Alegre: Artmed, 2012.

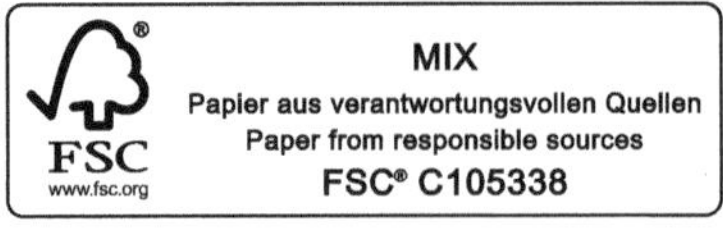

Printed by Books on Demand GmbH, Norderstedt / Germany